Japan's Dietary Transition and Its Impacts

Food, Health, and the Environment

Series Editor: Robert Gottlieb, Henry R. Luce Professor of Urban and Environmental Policy, Occidental College

Japan's Dietary Transition and Its Impacts

Vaclav Smil and Kazuhiko Kobayashi

The MIT Press
Cambridge, Massachusetts
London, England

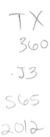
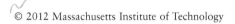
MIT Press books may be purchased at special quantity discounts for business or sales promotional use. For information, please email special_sales@mitpress.mit.edu or write to Special Sales Department, The MIT Press, 55 Hayward Street, Cambridge, MA 02142.

This book was set in Sabon by Toppan Best-set Premedia Limited. Printed and bound in the United States of America.

Library of Congress Cataloging-in-Publication Data

Smil, Vaclav.
Japan's dietary transition and its impacts / Vaclav Smil and Kazuhiko Kobayashi.
  p. cm.—(Food, health, and the environment)
Includes bibliographical references and index.
ISBN 978-0-262-01782-4 (hardcover : alk. paper)
1. Diet—Japan—Longitudinal studies. 2. Food habits—Japan—Longitudinal studies. 3. Diet—Health aspects—Japan. 4. Food consumption forecasting—Japan. 5. Agricultural ecology—Japan. I. Kobayashi, Kazuhiko, 1946– II. Title
TX360.J3S65 2012
641.5′630952—dc23
2011053214

10 9 8 7 6 5 4 3 2 1

Contents

Series Foreword

I am pleased to present the ninth book in the Food, Health, and the Environment series. This series explores the global and local dimensions of food systems and examines issues of access, justice, and environmental and community well-being. It includes books that focus on the way food is grown, processed, manufactured, distributed, sold, and consumed. Among the matters addressed are what foods are available to communities and individuals, how those foods are obtained, and what health and environmental factors are embedded in food system choices and outcomes. The series focuses not only on food security and well-being but also on regional, state, national, and international policy decisions and economic and cultural forces. Food, Health, and the Environment books provide a window into the public debates, theoretical considerations, and multidisciplinary perspectives that have made food systems and their connections to health and environment important subjects of study.

Robert Gottlieb, Occidental College
Series editor

Preface

This book is about long-term dietary change and its consequences for agricultural production, trade, food consumption, environment, and health. Its scope dictates interdisciplinary coverage and precludes any simple categorization: the book draws on findings from historical and economic studies, agronomic and agricultural analyses, and the fields of nutrition, public health, demography, and environmental science. The intent has been to present a multifaceted evaluation of a process whose nature and impact can be truly appreciated only through a broad-based inquiry. At the same time, this means that the book will disappoint if it is judged from narrow perspectives of specific expertise: it is not an exercise in economic history, nutritional science, or agricultural development.

Dietary transition—a gradual shift from traditional, preindustrial diets dominated by plant foods to a new pattern of intakes that includes more animal foodstuffs, more fats, more sugar, and a greater variety of processed foods—has been a universal phenomenon, but Japan offers a particularly interesting illustration of the process with several unique characteristics. The country's dietary transition was a key ingredient of its modernization that made it the world's second largest economic power of the second half of the twentieth century. Although the transition began slowly during the Meiji era (1868–1912), it proceeded at remarkably rapid rates once the country repaired the massive wartime damage by the mid-1950s, and most of it was subsequently accomplished in just a single generation, a tempo that has been rivaled only recently in urban China.

But perhaps its most remarkable attribute has been its saturation at levels well below the spending potential of such an affluent society. After rising appreciably since World War II, the average Japanese per capita intakes of meat and dairy products, and even more so those of fats and sugar, have remained much below the means that prevail in high-income Western countries. There is no doubt that this profound and yet limited change of diet has been a key factor in propelling Japan to its enviable demographic primacy—the country has had the world's highest life expectancy since the mid-1960s—and making its population generally healthier and by far the least overweight or obese among all modern affluent countries.

The two most notable costs of these achievements, Japan's high dependence on food imports and environmental impacts of intensive food production, also have important global implications. No other affluent country imports as much of its food supply (recently about 60 percent on food energy basis) as Japan does. Even in absolute terms, Japan is the world's largest importer of cereals, recently buying about four times as much as China, largely the result of its huge purchases of feed corn, as well as of pork and (in terms of overall value) seafood. Obviously Japan's food trade has an effect on the worldwide price of these major commodities. And these imports also mean that more farmland is used to grow Japan's food and feed crops abroad (particularly in the U.S. Corn Belt) and that the environmental impacts of irrigation and intensive use of nitrogenous fertilizers are felt more in food-exporting countries. The environmental impacts have been also felt in the ocean: Japan's massive imports of seafood, and particularly of fish species at the top of marine food webs, have exerted a strong worldwide impact on marine biota.

As a result, we think that these realities of more than a century of gradual but profound dietary changes with major domestic and foreign implications are of interest to many readers. That is why we have written a book that we hope can be read with some profit by nonspecialists who seek reliable information about a remarkable historical, economic, social, and nutritional phenomenon, as well as by various specialists who may find little new in their fields of expertise but may profit from finding some useful connections, links, and conclusions in other fields. The book's scope dictates its progression, with the focus first on the composition of Japan's food consumption and on its long-term changes (chapters 1 through 3) and, second, on the consequences of this process–first on the nation's health and longevity (chapter 4) and then on the key environmental impacts of Japan's intensive agriculture and high level of food and feed imports (chapter 5).

The first two chapters deal with the basics of Japanese diet. They go over a ground that is familiar to many experts on Japanese food, diets, agriculture, and economic history but that must be revisited for the benefit of more or less uninitiated readers who need first to understand the composition of the country's traditional diets in order to appreciate their modern transformation. Chapter 3 looks at this transformation from the perspective of dietary transition studies, explaining the process in terms of changing food energy supply and intakes and shifting shares of nutrients. Chapter 4 offers interdisciplinary syntheses of the transition's effects on health and longevity, and chapter 5 examines its impacts on land, water, nitrogen flows, and marine biota in Japan and abroad. Chapter 6 sums up the record and offers a few comments about future options. As far as we know, no other book provides such a comparably systematic and broad coverage of these diverse consequences.

One attribute common to all chapters is their strongly quantitative aspect. Historical trends are best followed with numbers: true appreciation of changes and a realistic understanding of what has been accomplished and what may lie ahead come only from detailed quantitative appraisals. That is why the book does not skimp on numbers; undoubtedly some readers will think that they are too many. Making the book strongly quantitative has been possible thanks to Japan's unusual wealth of historical and modern statistics, but this abundance also presents a problem. With so much statistical information filling the book in order to explain, illustrate, and quantify a century of economic, agricultural, population, dietary, trade, energy, and environmental changes and with so many factual explanations needed to familiarize Western readers with many details of Japanese foodways, it would be distracting to reference every number and every fact mentioned in the text. Instead, we offer here a short list of key references that we used to extract the relevant data and confirm many facts. Beyond these, the book contains hundreds of other specific references that offer more detailed examination of every major subject we treat here.

Japan has some of the world's most comprehensive, and highly reliable, series of historical statistics and these materials were conveniently compiled in a multivolume series edited by Ōkawa, Shinohara, and

Umemura (1987–1988). This series was later extended and expanded, and its online bilingual version now contains 879 statistical tables in 31 categories ranging from land and climate to environment and defense (Statistics Bureau 2011a). All historical statistics are taken from these sources, and the latest data have been extracted from Japan's statistical yearbook (Statistics Bureau 2011b) or from the periodical publications of the Ministry of Health, Labor, and Welfare dealing with agricultural production, fisheries, national food balance sheets, and surveys of nutrition intake.

Information on economy, agriculture, and life during the late Tokugawa period (1603–1868) in general, and on the capital (Edo) and its culinary culture in particular, can be found in Dunn (1969), Harada (1989, 2008), Hanley (1997), Nishiyama (1997), Ishige (2001) and Rath (2010). The twentieth-century history of changes in Japanese agriculture is covered in King (1911), Nakamura (1966), Ōkawa, Johnston, and Kaneda (1970), Ogura (1980), Hayami (1988), Van der Meer and Yamada (1990), and Hayami and Yamada (1991). Japanese foodways, meal ingredients, cooking techniques, and culinary lore are described and explained in Tsuji (1980), Richie (1985), Hosking (1996), Davidson (1999), Ishige (2000, 2001), Ashkenazi and Jacob (2000), Cwiertka (2007), and Rath and Assmann (2010).

For those eager to prepare Japanese dishes, there is no shortage of well-informed and well-illustrated sources. Notable contributions include books by Tsuji (1980; the latest edition was published in 2007), Yoneda and Hoshino (1998), Kazuko (2001), Kurihara (2006), Morimoto (2007), and Arimoto (2010). The latest food news can be followed in *Japan Food Trends*, published by the Global Agriculture Information Network of the U.S. Department of Agriculture's Foreign Agricultural Service in Tokyo (GAIN 2011) and on the Trends in Japan Web site (http://web-japan.org/trends).

Finally, we give all Japanese names in the text in the Western order, with first name preceding surname, and we transcribe all Japanese words by using revised Hepburn *rōmaji* and set them in italics (tofu and sushi, now commonly used worldwide, and the names of large cities being the only exceptions).

Abbreviations

kcal	kilocalories
kcal/capita	kilocalories per capita
kg	kilograms
kg/capita	kilograms per capita
km	kilometers
m^2	square meters
m^2/capita	square meters per capita
mg N/L	micrograms of nitrogen per liter
Mha	million hectares
Mt	million tonnes (metric tons)

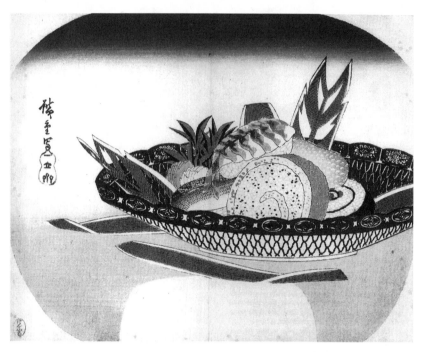

A classic portrayal of Japan's most famous meal: Andō Hiroshige's 1843 *ukiyo-e* plate of sushi containing both *nigirizushi* (gizzard shad, *kohada*, on the left, shrimp, *ebi*, on the top) and *makizushi* (rolls wrapped in *tamago* and *nori*).

1

Japanese Diet, 1900–2010: From Subsistence to Affluence

During the 1970s, Junichi Saga began recording the memories of his patients, who were born mostly during the last decade of the nineteenth and the first decade of the twentieth century and lived in, or near, Tsuchiura, in the Lake Kasumigaura region. Almost uniformly, those testimonies depict diets that were at or barely above basic subsistence level, with rice scarce, with high consumption of less preferred barley, and with animal protein almost entirely absent. Here are the recollections of Ihara Orinosuke, born in 1904 (Saga 1987, 187): "In our village a meal of a mixture of rice and barley, with six parts barley to four parts rice, would've been considered above average. . . . Fresh river fish we almost never had up in the mountain where I lived. . . . We never saw any fresh sea fish, either, from one year to the next. But at New Year most families bought one salted salmon, though only after an awful fuss."

And even when the relatively better-off townspeople needed animal protein for a sick person, they had little choice but to go to outcasts (*sanka*) who used to kill and eat wild dogs (Saga 1987, 51): "In those days even low-class meat such as horse or rabbit was almost impossible to get hold of, so when, for instance, someone was ill and needed extra protein, even townspeople would be forced to go along and buy some dogmeat from the *sanka*." And this was half a century after Japan began its determined modernization drive, and in an area only some 60 km northeast of downtown Tokyo and 40 km from the nearest Pacific shoreline.

Prevalence of poor subsistence diets reported by Saga's patients is confirmed by Japan's historical statistics (Statistics Bureau 2011a). Even on a nationwide scale, rice production in 1900 was only about three times the amount of harvested barley, but then the ratio began to rise, and by 2010, it reached roughly 40:1. In 1900 nationwide pork production prorated to a minuscule amount of less than 30 grams a year per capita, which means that in reality, most people never ate any pork. Virtually no poultry was produced for meat, a heritage of medieval *shintō* taboos that saw fowl as announcers of dawn rather than a source of food (Ishige 2000). Egg production averaged only one egg per person every month, and the country, which had no tradition of consuming dairy products, produced annually less than half a teaspoon of milk per capita: more than 99 percent of Japanese population never drank any milk.

A century later, few countries can rival Japan in the quality of its diet (FAO 2011a). At the beginning of the twenty-first century, Japan was producing annually about 20 kg of meat per capita and importing even more than that for a total annual per capita supply of about 45 kg; its per capita milk production reached 65 liters, and imports of dairy products boosted the total supply in terms of fluid milk to some 85 liters, while seafood availability came close to 60 kg per capita (about half of it imported), the highest consumption of marine food worldwide. All of these rates represent huge gains—in relative terms, far higher than comparable twentieth-century gains in the United States and Europe, where consumption of animal foods was fairly high as early as 1900. The growth of Japan's food supply is no less impressive in absolute terms, especially when taking into account the intervening population increase, from fewer than 44 million in 1900 to more than 126 million by the year 2000, or nearly a tripling of the nationwide count in a century.

The food balance sheets of the Food and Agricultural Organization (FAO 2011a) show that in the year 2000, average per capita availability of food was significantly lower in Japan (about 2,800 kcal per day) than in the major economies of the European Union (about 3,500 kcal per day) or the United States (nearly 3,800 kcal per day) but those differences were not a sign of any inferior diet, merely of a less wasteful consumption. As far as the actual food consumption was concerned, Japan's annual dietary surveys—whose detail and continuity have no counterpart in any other affluent economy—indicated daily average of about 1,950 kcal per capita in the year 2000 (Statistics Bureau 2011a), compared to about 2,100 kcal per capita in the United States (Wright et al. 2003). In food energy terms, the difference in actual consumption was thus less than 10 percent: the U.S. and Japanese consumption means were nearly identical for carbohydrates and were less than 15 percent apart for all proteins, but they differed by about 40 percent for dietary fats, a reality that is not of any health benefit for Americans.

Nutrition has critical roles in child development, and prevailing diets have obvious (albeit complex and in many ways contentious) associations with the prevalence of a healthy and active adult life, with relatively disease-free aging, and with the longevity of populations. Japanese historical statistics clearly show the role of diet in development, with the average height of 10 year old boys rising from 123.9 centimeters in 1900 to 139.1 centimeters a century later, roughly a 12 percent gain. And perhaps no other indicator of the overall adequacy and quality of Japanese diet is more impressive than the country's still improving record of average life expectancy. Japanese women rose to the top of the global longevity ranking in 1985 when their average life expectancy at birth surpassed 80 years (80.48), and men joined them a year later when their average life expectancy exceeded 75 years (Ministry of Health and Welfare 1995). A quarter-century later, both sexes continue to hold this primacy, with Japanese female expectancy now at roughly 86 years and the male mean at just above 79 years (Statistics Bureau 2011a). Obviously better nutrition was not the only factor explaining the gains in body growth and longevity: advances in public health and overall gains in the quality of life were other key contributors.

The story of Japan's dietary transition is even more remarkable because most of the qualitative gains have been achieved only since the early 1950s, after the country emerged from the destruction of World War II and from difficult years of postwar reconstruction: Japan's highest prewar gross domestic product, reached in 1939, was not equaled until 1953 (Okawa, Ito and Noda 1957; Statistics Bureau 2011a). And thanks to a relatively large amounts of mostly good-quality historical statistics (some of them available in series stretching over a century, and nearly all of them complete for the post-1950 period), the country's dietary transition, and its multifaceted repercussions, can be studied in many revealing details.

In chapter 2, we take a close, systematic look at the changing consumption of individual foodstuffs, ranging from a gradual retreat of some traditional staples to a rapid adoption of foods that were never (or very rarely) consumed in preindustrial (or pre–World War II) Japan. In chapter 3 we quantify these long-term dietary transformations in terms of average food supply (relying on food balance sheets) and average food consumption (based on Japan's unique household surveys and tracing actual consumption of food energy and individual macronutrients) and explain the continuity and change in Japan's still rather unique dietary pattern. We first review the associations between the Japanese diet (focusing on its special characteristics) and the nation's exceptional longevity and incidence of major diseases and then close with an examination of Japanese foodways in long-term perspective, pointing out both rapid changes and notable continuities and describing their impact on foreign food and beverage choices.

Chapter 4 focuses on the environmental impact of Japan's dietary transitions. Those great gains in the quality of Japanese diet have exacted their price in terms of land use changes and water requirements, widespread intensification of crop production has resulted in rising losses of reactive nitrogen (due to enormous increases in the use of nitrogenous fertilizers), and more aggressive, as well as more wide-ranging, exploitation of marine resources has been an important contributor to the excessive exploitation of many fish and invertebrate species. And because Japan is more dependent on food and feed imports than any other large modern economy, environmental impacts of those imports must be considered alongside the changes that have taken place in the country and within its coastal waters. That is why we also examine virtual land, water, and nutrient needs embodied in products shipped from abroad.

Many of these environmental changes are strongly and dynamically intertwined. For example, land use change due to the expansion of flooded fields to produce more rice also has inevitable consequences for water management and fertilizer use, with higher nitrogen inputs leading to greater leaching and denitrification losses—and abandoning paddy fields, eating less rice, and consuming more meat triggers a chain of environmental consequences that can extend to several continents because of rising imports of corn and soybeans from the United States and Brazil and preparation of fish-based feeds from species caught in African waters. We call attention to these linkages, but a systematic appraisal of environmental impacts caused by Japan's remarkable dietary transition is done best by a sequential examination of its key components.

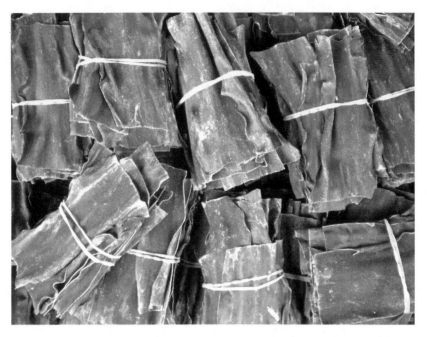

An old and quintessentially Japanese foodstuff that remains in favor: bundles of dried seaweed (kelp, *konbu*) to be used in preparing *dashi*, the essential stock of Japan's cuisine. (V. Smil)

2
Old and New Foodstuffs: A Century of Transitions

There is no shortage of universal, nearly universal, or very common trends that unfolded across the eventful twentieth century. Entries on this list could range from unprecedented growth of populations to no less unprecedented rates of urbanization, from economic integration and globalization to the advances in electronic communication and information, from the spread of democracy to the countertrend of political extremism, and from consumerism and mass affluence to weakened governance and fiscal mismanagement. But it is not very likely that any such list prepared by historians, economists, and students of political and military affairs and technical advances would include a critical trend that has been improving the quality of life for billions of people while also changing entire economic sectors and trading patterns and affecting (too often negatively) the environment on scales ranging from local to global.

This virtually universal trend of a fundamental importance and of far-reaching consequences is known as dietary transition—but *dietary* (or *nutritional*) *transformation* might be an equally good term. Its trajectory is obvious: from traditional diets of overwhelmingly rural societies to modern diets of largely urban populations in affluent postindustrial economies (in North America, Europe, Japan, and Australia), as well as in still rapidly modernizing nations, and above all in China, India, Indonesia, and Brazil (Bengoa 2001; Caballero and Popkin 2002; Lee 2002; Shetty 2002; Lipoeto et al. 2004; Smil 2004; Weng and Caballero 2007). The only countries where this transformation is yet to unfold (or where it is in its earliest stages and restricted to better-off urban areas) are the poorest nations of sub-Saharan Africa and the least developed states in Asia (Afghanistan, Laos, Nepal).

Principal components of dietary transition have been remarkably uniform around the world. On one hand, there is a declining consumption of traditional starchy carbohydrate staples (cereal grains as well as tubers) and usually an even faster declining demand for legumes (all key sources of protein in preindustrial diets); on the other hand there is rising consumption of all kinds of animal foods (meat, fish, eggs, dairy products) and growing demand for a greater variety and a better quality of fruits and vegetables. While staple carbohydrate foods provided at least two-thirds (and often over four-fifths) of all food energy in preindustrial societies, their share in modern diets is mostly below one-third, with minima just around one-quarter. Declines in coarse grain consumption are almost invariably more pronounced as corn, barley, buckwheat, millets, oats, and rye yield to, or are displaced by, rice and wheat.

At the same time, more corn is grown than ever before (or imported) for animal feed, and the same is true for soybeans. As a result, direct consumption of wheat and rice is being displaced by higher indirect intakes of corn and soybeans used as the most efficient feeds for rising production of meat, eggs, and milk. Rising incomes create higher demand not only for meat and eggs but also, though less universally, for fish and milk, and this leads to a rapid decline in consumption of protein-rich legumes (soybeans, common beans, lentils, chickpeas). Other notable components are greater consumption of processed foods and carbonated beverages and, hence, higher average intakes of sugars and fats.

Although diets with an increasing amount of meat are a universal component of dietary transition, their specific composition varies considerably due to national production (countries with limited area of farmland and grassland cannot produce much beef), affordability of imports (frozen poultry is much less expensive than fresh beef), and food taboos and dietary preferences (Muslim proscription of pork, Hindu avoidance of beef, widespread abstention from eating horse meat). And traditional food preferences and income levels also determine the pace of this transition and its eventual saturation levels. Annual meat supply in Spain, as in other countries adhering to a traditional low-meat Mediterranean diet, was less than 20 kg/capita during the late 1950s, but it more than tripled in a single generation and rose to more than 100 kg/capita by the year 2000 to become one of Europe's highest, surpassing both the French and German rates (Food and Agriculture Organization 2011a). In contrast, Japan still prefers to import more seafood than meat.

A complete list of foodstuffs consumed by any traditional society contained scores of items ranging from plant roots and invertebrate animals all the way to large terrestrial mammals and just about any kind of marine organisms. Thanks to a high biodiversity of its forests and coastal waters, pre-Buddhist Japan was an excellent example of this eclectic eating that was not circumscribed by any dietary taboos: wild animals were hunted, and eating of wild plants, fish, and aquatic invertebrates supplemented food from cultivated crops. Some of those ancient traditions persist in modern Japan. Appreciation of foodstuffs that are available only in specific seasons and fondness for wild herbs and vegetables (*sansai* as opposed to the cultivated *yasai*) are notable examples of this persistence. Specific parts of numerous species of wild plants— ranging from ostrich fern fiddleheads (*kogomi*) to unopened buds of Japanese butterbur (*fukinotō*)—are still the basis of a special (and now often very expensive) vegetarian cuisine (*sansai ryōri*). The wild plants are so popular that some of them are now cultivated and thus the border between cultivated and wild plants has become blurred.

The Buddhist proscription of animal killing led to increasingly stringent bans on eating animal foods, although fish and other marine species were always exempt from this proscription and a highly inventive temple-based Buddhist vegetarian cuisine (*shōjin ryōri*) came up with a variety of meat substitutes using tofu and *fu*, or wheat gluten (Yoneda and Hoshino 1998). But even as the range of foodstuffs commonly consumed during the Tokugawa (or Edo) era (1603–1868) was reduced compared to the situation that prevailed in medieval Japan, some species introduced during the Western presence in Japan since the mid-sixteenth century (most notably potato, sweet potato, peppers, squashes, corn, melon, spinach) persisted in the country's fields after the country's rulers cut off any further exchanges with Europe except for a tiny Dutch presence at Deshima. In particular, corn, potato, and sweet potato had spread widely in the upland fields during the Tokugawa era and supported the population in mountains and islands, where rice paddies could hardly be developed.

Dietary innovations and returns to abandoned traditions that took place during the Meiji era had only a limited impact on common diets: bread could be bought in newly established bakeries in major cities, but an overwhelming majority of peasants would never taste it. The emperor himself approved of eating beef, but that meat was beyond reach of all but those belonging to small urban Westernizing elites; elements of Western cuisine (*yōshoku*) began to be accepted in a few major urban areas (Tokyo, Yokohama, Osaka, and Kobe), but an overwhelming majority of Japan's rural and small town population (in 1900, cities with more than 10,000 people accounted still for no less than 20 percent of the country's inhabitants) continued the frugal Japanese cuisine whose norms were set during the thirteen generations of the Tokugawa era.

And once even the common everyday diets began to change—slowly around the end of the nineteenth century, more perceptibly during the interwar years, and then rather rapidly after the country emerged from its postwar poverty during mid-1950s—the most important shifts and the most consequential impacts concerned the staple foodstuffs. In its fundamentals, Japan's dietary transition has not been unique or highly unusual, but because it has affected every major food category, its key features can be captured only by tracing the changes in every one of a half-dozen major food groups: carbohydrate staples (cereals and tubers), legumes, vegetables and fruits, seafood, meat, and dairy products.

Carbohydrate Staples

No traditional diet could be dependent on a single carbohydrate staple; that would have been both a costly and very risky strategy given the different growing requirements of crops and the unpredictable fluctuations of weather-dependent harvests. In Europe (and particularly in the continent's northern half), wheat was not the only staple cereal grain: rye, oats, barley, and buckwheat were widely cultivated, and they were often as important ingredients in commonly consumed breads as was wheat. After their introduction from South America, potatoes became another indispensable starchy staple in countries from Ireland to Poland and from France to Russia. China had always relied on millets, wheat, and rice, supplemented by soybeans and various beans, and a similar situation applied in India where both the northern reliance on wheat and millets and the southern preference for rice were accompanied by unusually high intakes of legumes (above all, lentils).

In premodern Japan, short-grained rice—*Oryza sativa* var. *japonica*; growing rice *ine*, rice grains *kome*, harvested brown, unmilled (unpolished) grains *genmai*, cooked rice *meshi or gohan*—was never the only

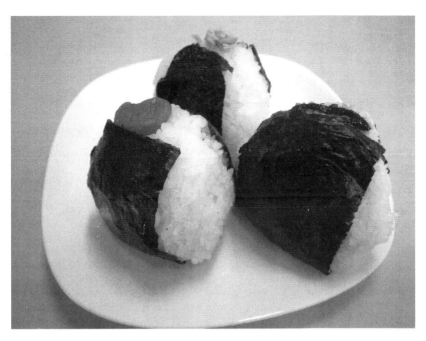

Figure 2.1
Although rice has ceased to be the dominant staple, the grain is still eaten widely. Rice balls (*onigiri* or *omusubi*), wrapped in *nori* and often flavored with a pickled Japanese apricot (*umeboshi*), remain a favorite snack. (K. Kobayashi)

staple. The other carbohydrate staples included millets—*awa* (foxtail millet), *kibi* (proso millet), *morokoshi* (Indian millet) and *hie* (barnyard millet)—barley (*ōmugi*), wheat (*komugi*, and buckwheat (*soba*). Mixtures of these grains (in the poorest regions and during famine years with hardly any rice included) were served in various ways. For example, barley grains were roughly ground and boiled with rice to be served as *mugi-meshi*. Vegetables, whether collected or cultivated, were often mixed with rice to make *kate-meshi*. Making the grains into porridges (*kayu*) or *zōsui*—grains boiled in soup with vegetables—was a common practice to save precious grains while filling the stomachs. Rice grains of poor quality were ground with other grains and made into dumplings to be boiled in soup. In some regions, ground grains were baked slowly in the hearth to produce *yakimochi* or *oyaki*, a kind of unleavened bread (Hanley 1997). Beginning in the seventeenth century, potatoes and sweet potatoes were added.

Rice

People of all classes always preferred rice, and eventually highly milled white rice, but only those who were well-off could afford it regularly during the early Tokugawa years. The famous Keian edict of 1649 (*Keian no ofuregaki,* cited here in translation in Ooms 1996) admonishes peasants for their common "lack of judgment" because they "do not think ahead; hence they carelessly feed their wives and children rice and other grains when these are harvested in the fall, but they should always take as good care of food as they do in the first, second, and third [winter] months of the year." The edict is clear that diets should be frugal and that rice should be consumed only in moderation:

Wheat, foxtail millet, barnyard grass, greens, radishes, and any other grains should be planted so that rice is not depleted by eating it in great quantities. . . . Everybody, from the house owner down to his children and servants, and so on, should normally eat plain food. However, at times of demanding labor, like planting rice seedlings or harvesting, slightly better food should be made available in large amounts. If one shows such consideration regarding food, everyone will be content and work hard.

Fragmentary testimonies in descriptions of daily life, diaries and, later, a few actual consumption surveys available for some regions (Shinano, Satsuma, Chōshū) during the eighteenth and the early nineteenth centuries show complex consumption patterns that were determined by a combination of social class, income, location, and harvest. Most people did eat some rice at least once a day, but they continued to subsist on grain mixtures supplemented by legumes, sweet potatoes, vegetables, and wild plants, and their diets showed notable seasonal fluctuations in both quantity and quality. At one extreme were the best-off samurai families who ate polished rice several times a day. And at the other end of the nutritional spectrum were peasants in the poorest mountainous regions who had to buy rice from the lowland producers and could afford it only as an occasional treat.

During the last century of the Tokugawa rule, as incomes rose and growing cities offered greater food choices to their better-off inhabitants, urban diets showed some notable changes. Consumption of highly polished white rice (available only since the beginning of the eighteenth century due to the changes in milling) began to spread, numerous cookbooks were published, many new restaurants, particularly those serving *soba* noodles, sushi, and freshwater eels (*unagi*), were opened, and eating out became a custom for many urbanites, including those who were far from rich. There are many indications that urban residents ate rice three times a day by the middle of the Edo period (1603–1868). Nevertheless, the combination of grains (albeit it with more, and more polished, rice) remained the dominant source of Japan's food energy and most of its protein and micronutrients. On the last score, those who could afford to eat white rice were unknowingly inflicting on themselves a major micronutrient deficiency, beriberi, resulting in a painful physical and neural deterioration leading to fatal heart failure, due to a chronic shortage of vitamin B1 (thiamine) that was previously readily obtainable in brown rice bran (Carpenter 2000).

The changes ushered in as Japan opened to the West during the first decades of the Meiji era (1868–1912) were more discernible in some rapid adoption of Western technical innovations and even first domestic inventions (Morris-Suzuki 1994) rather than in everyday diets. Indeed, a case can be made (supported by official statistics whose accuracy for the earliest Meiji decades is questionable but whose quality had improved with time) that the basic dietary pattern of the last Tokugawa decades persevered with only a few minor shifts during the early Meiji period. In 1867, the earliest year for which comparative crop statistics are available, rice accounted for about 47 percent of main staple foodstuffs, barley for about 28 percent, and other cereals for roughly 19 percent; two decades later, the share for rice was up to nearly 60 percent, barley down to 16 percent, other cereals declined to less than 5 percent, and potatoes made up the remainder (Bassino 2006).

This confirms a little appreciated fact that rice, ancient as its cultivation is in Japan, became the country's indisputably dominant primary staple crop (both in terms of quantity consumed and perception of quotidian indispensability) only in the not-so-distant past. According to Tsukuba (1986) and Ōmameuda (2007), it became a truly dominant staple for the majority of population only during the Meiji era. Dore (1958) thought that white rice became part of the Japanese birthright only during the 1930s, and Watanabe (1989) went even further, stating that rice became the staple only in 1939 with the advent of food rationing. In any case, rice had a prominent place in the nation's cosmology, identity, self-perception, and culture for centuries before it became an indispensable staple. Many works examine the meaning of rice as a symbol of wealth, power, and beauty and its many metaphoric, historic, environmental, communal, and aesthetic attributes. Ohnuki-Tierney (1993) offers an excellent review of all major Japanese writings on this often emotionally charged topic. A closer look at the twentieth-century trends in major components of the Japanese diet must then start with the supply of rice.

In 1900 paddy rice accounted for nearly 55 percent of all cultivated area, and its harvest was almost twice as large as the combined harvest of all other cereal (wheat, barley, buckwheat) and leguminous (soybeans, beans) grains, and it accounted for about 60 percent of all food energy available in plant foods. There are disagreements regarding the average rice yields during the early years of the Meiji era, mainly because of likely underregistration of land and underreporting of yields (Mosk 1978; Bassino 2006)—but there is no doubt that at the beginning of the twentieth century, Japan's traditional rice cropping had already reached high levels of productivity based solely on animate labor and the use of organic fertilizers.

In 1900 the average yield of husked rice was about 2.25 tonnes per hectare, by 1940 it was just short of 3 tonnes per hectare, and postwar improvements in plant breeding, agronomic management and nutrient supply lifted the mean above 4 tonnes per hectare by the late 1960s; the century ended with harvests averaging about 5.0 to 5.4 tonnes per hectare (table 2.1). Initially, these gains relied on highly labor-intensive cropping (as many as 300 days per hectare in the early 1900s and still as many as 200 days by 1940), but after the war, mechanization of fieldwork and the switch from organic to synthetic fertilizers reduced the inputs to just 500 hours per hectare by 1990 (International Rice Research Institute 2009a). Although the average yield of Japanese paddy rice rose 2.4 times during the twentieth century, that rate was lower than the 2.9-fold increase of the country's population.

But this difference did not create any supply shortages, and after World War II, when the absolute population growth was greater than before the war (28 million between 1900 and 1940, 33 million between 1950 and 1990), it did not require any imports. Small-scale (equal to 1 to 3 percent of total consumption) rice imports began during the 1870s, but it was only between 1920 and 1940, when the country's population expanded at roughly twice the rate, that the supply-demand situation became very

Table 2.1
Rice production and supply, 1900–2008

Year	Planted area (Mha)	Harvest (Mt)	Yield (t/ha)	Net imports[a] (Mt)	Supply[b] (Mt)	Average annual supply[c] (kg/capita)
1900	2.81	6.22	2.21	0.11	6.33	144
1925	3.13	8.96	2.86	1.01	9.97	167
1935	3.18	8.61	2.71	1.83	10.44	151
1950	3.01	9.65	3.21	0.72	10.37	123
1965	3.26	12.41	3.81	1.05	13.00	131
1975	2.76	13.17	4.77	—	12.00	107
1990	2.07	10.50	5.07	—	10.50	85
2000	1.77	9.49	5.36	0.40	9.79	77
2008	1.63	8.82	5.41	0.70	8.86	69

a. Denotes quantities of less than 0.1 Mt.
b. Totals take into account annual changes in stocks.
c. All values are rounded to the nearest kilogram and refer to unmilled (paddy) rice.

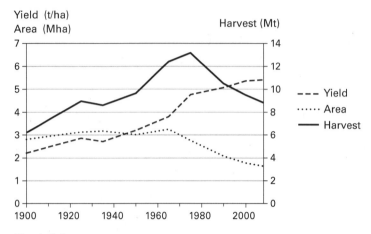

Graph 2.1
Rice planted area, yield, and harvest for 1900–2008.

tight and the country had to import considerable quantities of rice (as much as 19 percent of the total supply in 1935) from Taiwan and Korea, its two Asian colonies (Ogura1980; Ōmameuda 2007; see also table 2.1). But as soon as the production recovered from the postwar lows, the rising yields easily satisfied the growing demand, output peaked during the late 1960s at about 14.5 Mt per year and then began its still continuing decline that brought it to just 9 Mt by 2005 (table 2.1; graph 2.1).

When expressed in per capita terms, Japan's average supply of unhusked rice was almost 140 kg per year during the first decade of the twentieth century, by 1920 it surpassed 160 kg, and by 1940 it declined to about 125 kg/capita. In 1945 the supply (at 80 kg/capita) was at a near-starvation level, and although it recovered to 120 kg in 1946, it remained precarious until the early 1950s. Japan's post-1950 supply of rice can be divided into three distinct periods. First was the time of unmet demand and rising production that brought new absolute consumption and production peaks (in 1963 and 1967). This temporary increase of staple grain demand is a common feature of an early stage of modern dietary transition when rising incomes go first to buy full satiation levels of traditional staples. In Japan's case, this common trend was catalyzed by the fact that the beginnings of prosperity came so quickly after a period of wartime and postwar food shortages.

The second period was characterized by a relatively rapid decline of per capita demand and surplus domestic production without any imports

(1968–1995). Subsequently Japan has experienced abundant supply as its falling domestic output has been supplemented by imports due to trade liberalization. Average annual per capita rice supply rose from 120 kg in 1946 (when it still provided about 60 percent of all food energy) to just over 130 kg by 1960, when its food energy share fell below 50 percent and it cost an average household nearly a quarter of its total food expenditure and a tenth of its overall outlays. Subsequent uninterrupted decline of demand, with the fastest decrements between 1965 and 1975 and at a slower pace ever since, brought the average per capita supply of milled rice to just above 60 kg per year by 2000 when rice provided less than a quarter of all food energy, less than animal products and fats.

Most of the harvested rice (as much as 95 percent during the preindustrial era and 88 percent in recent years) has been eaten as white polished grain (*hakumai*) prepared by boiling in water to yield cooked rice (*gohan* or *meshi*). After milling, the typical extraction rate is 73 percent compared to the preferred rates of as low as 65 percent in Vietnam and the Philippines (International Rice Research Institute 2008). In traditional meals the dominant *gohan* is always accompanied by a variety of less voluminous side dishes (*okazu*), or it is eaten with green tea poured over it (*ochazuke*) and various toppings. *Gohan* is also eaten cold at any time of the day as snack food, typically in the form of rounded tetrahedron-shaped rice balls (*onigiri*) made of rice alone or wrapped in *nori* or filled with ingredients that contrast with bland *gohan*. The remainder of the harvested rice is processed to make *saké* and *miso* (more on these later in this chapter), soft and sticky rice cakes (*mochi*, made from special, glutinous varieties of rice, *mochigome*), rice crackers (*sembei, arare*), and other foodstuffs. Poor-quality rice unfit for sale has been used to make rice flour cakes, but unlike in China, Vietnam, or Thailand, Japanese rice has rarely been used for making translucent rice noodles.

Average per capita consumption of rice, 320 to 330 grams per day before the war, reached peaks of more than 360 grams per day in 1956, 1959, and 1961. By 1989 consumption dropped to less than 200 grams per day, and by 2000, they were just above 160 grams per day. Shares of rice in Japan's average food consumption show remarkable consistency for more than 100 years, since the beginning of the Meiji era to the early 1970s. Consumption surveys from the years 1870, 1880, and 1886 show that rice accounted for, respectively, about 50, 53, and 52 percent of all food energy and that barley was the second most important staple, with shares of 27 to 28 percent (Umemura, Takamatsu, and Itoh 1983). In 1950 the share was about 59 percent of all food energy, and its share peaked in 1959 with 62 percent; subsequent decline in demand brought the share to 40 percent by 1976.

Although consumption has declined, the Japanese still hold the milled grain in high regard. In January 2007 an Internet survey of more than 10,000 people found that rice remains a favorite staple of 75 percent of respondents (compared to just 9 percent of people preferring bread, 5 percent pasta, and just 1.5 percent *soba* (buckwheat noodles) and that 70 percent of them eat rice once or twice a day, 12 percent three or more times, and only 4 percent two to four times a week (MyVoice 2007). As for the preferences in eating and preparing rice, 55 percent said it must be domestically grown, a third insisted on white rice, and 12 percent chose brown rice. Five leading images of rice in the minds of respondents were "tasty," "never boring," "Japanese," "healthy," and "cannot live without it." But these professions of enduring fondness contrast with an undeniable fact that after more than a millennium as the dominant mainstay of Japanese civilization, rice has become just one of many increasingly affordable food choices and that an average household now spends less on its purchases than it does on buying bread and noodles. As Chern et al. (2003) put it, rice has ceased to be a staple food and become more of a luxury foodstuff.

Barley, Buckwheat, and Noodles
As in other Asian countries that have undergone dietary transition, Japan's falling consumption of rice has been accompanied by declining consumption of other traditional grains and by rising consumption of foodstuffs made from wheat flour—above all noodles, bread, and pastries. In Japan traditionally two kinds of coarse grains that were very important became marginalized by modernization: barley (ōmugi) and buckwheat (soba). In many poorer rural areas, barley was commonly mixed with rice to prepare staple steamed meals. Japan's barley harvest reached its first peak in 1913 (at about 2.4 Mt), it declined afterward, and its second peak, forty years later, was just a shade higher at nearly 2.6 Mt in 1954. Subsequent decline brought it to just 176,000 tonnes in 2000, and about 90 percent of barley used at that time in Japan (mainly in beer production) was imported.

Buckwheat was primarily eaten as a flour (*sobako*) to make a polenta-like porridge (*sobagaki*), dumplings (*sobadango*), and, on special occasions, buckwheat noodles (Udesky 1988). Most *soba* noodles sold in Japan now contain as much wheat flour as *sobako,* and sometimes more, but their favorite traditional serving as cold *zarusoba* has not changed. Japan's buckwheat harvest peaked in 1914 at about 150,000 tonnes and it was followed by an almost uninterrupted decline that brought it to only about 25,000 tonnes by 2000 when nearly 100,000 tonnes were imported (mostly from China, the United States, and Canada). This means that in 1914, per capita buckwheat supply averaged nearly 3 kg/capita, but in 2000 it was below 1 kg. Buckwheat noodles were the most popular food in the late Edo period—in 1860 the city had nearly 3,800 *soba* shops (*sobaya*), almost as many as today (Watanabe 2004)—and although they remain a favorite food, their per capita consumption is now less than a third of what it was nearly a century ago.

All other types of commonly eaten noodles (*menrui*) made of wheat flour were introduced from China between the twelfth and fourteenth centuries (Ito 2008): thick, soft, chewy, round strings of *udon*; thin, flat ribbons of *kishimen*; and the two kinds of vermicelli-like thin filaments that are sold dried only, *hiyamugi* and *sōmen.* Their postwar consumption expanded both due to more frequent choice of noodles at home and more noodle-serving establishments offering inexpensive, fast, and filling noodle dishes—but the Chinese-style noodles (*chūka soba or rāmen*, noodles served in a flavored stock with added slices of meat, seafood, or vegetables) did even better. *Rāmen* became popular first in Yokohama and Kobe, the two cities with large Chinese minorities, during the Meiji era. The Japanese fondness for noodles and increased interest in Chinese cuisine led to the proliferation of *rāmen* shops in some other cities, such as Tokyo and Sapporo, in the 1920s. But, it was only after World War II, with the many returnees from China, that *rāmen* became popular throughout Japan.

Such is the Japanese fondness for *rāmen* that when people were asked in a recent survey what food they would most like to eat after coming back home from a foreign trip, it came first, outranking such quintessentially Japanese meals as sushi, *onigiri,* and *miso shiru* (GOO 2007).

Instant *rāmen*—thin, pale, or yellowish, and often slightly curly wheat noodles prepared by a brief boiling or by steeping in a bowl or

disposable cup with added meat or vegetable flavors from a small sachet—
has become ubiquitous in Japan, Not only that, it has become one of
Japan's leading culinary exports to the West and, according to a poll
taken in 2000, nothing less than Japan's most important invention of the
twentieth century. Instant *rāmen* was introduced in August 1958 by Andō
Momofuku (born as Wu Baifu in Taiwan), the founder of Nissin Food
Products (Nissin Foods 2010; World Instant Noodles Association 2010).
His original recipe was to boil the noodles with a flavoring and then
remove nearly all the moisture by deep frying the noodles, a technique
previously used during the Qing dynasty, 1644–1912 in China, and
packing the dry noodles in individual serving portions.

Andō's basic production method is still the preferred way to make
instant *rāmen*. Wheat flour, starch, gluten, water, and salt (plus assorted
antioxidants, stabilizers, and preservatives) are used to make dough that
is cut into noodles (straight or wavy), which are then dried by frying for
one to two minutes in oil at 140°C to 160°C in order to reduce their
moisture to just 2 to 5 percent (hot drying not using oil is also possible,
but it makes it more difficult to achieve uniform product, the noodles
spoil more easily, and they require a longer cooking time). When Nissin
introduced its instant *rāmen*, fresh noodles were much less expensive, and
retailers saw little prospect for the dried product. But the three-minute
noodles had an enthusiastic public acceptance, and many companies
began to compete for an expanding market. In 1971 Nissin introduced
its even more successful Cup Noodles in a container. Scores of different
flavors became available in Asia and beyond: the United States is now
their fourth largest consumer, behind China, Indonesia, and Japan.

According to the World Instant Noodle Association (2010), global
retail sales in 2008 approached 100 billion packets (bags or cups). Not
surprisingly, China was in the lead (consuming nearly half of the total,
about 45 billion units), and in relative terms South Korea was number
one, with nearly 70 per capita servings a year, ahead of Japan's 40 units
per capita. Total output of Japanese instant noodles now approaches 1.3
Mt per year, with Nissin Food Products firmly in the lead (with some 30
percent of the market), followed by Tōyō Suisan (about 15 percent), and
Sanyō Foods (almost 10 percent).

Consumption of Italian pasta will never come close to that of Chinese-
and Japanese-style noodles, but more than 250,000 tonnes of it are now

consumed annually in Japan, with Nisshin Seifun and Nippon Seifun the leading producers, and with nearly half of the total consumption imported, primarily from Italy. In 2007 Japanese per capita pasta consumption was 21 servings (100 grams each) compared to about 70 servings in the United States and 280 in Italy.

Bread

The other most important reason for rising wheat consumption has been a relatively widespread adoption of leavened bread, for millennia the dominant staple of nearly all European diets. But bread was unknown in ancient Japan, and when it was introduced by the Portuguese in 1543 (hence *pan*, from the Portuguese *pão*), it failed to make any inroads. Gradual acceptance began only after the Meiji restoration. As elsewhere, its adoption has been facilitated by its convenience in preparing snacks, rapid urbanization (13 percent of Japan's population were urban in 1900, nearly 25 percent by 1930, almost 45 percent by 1960, and 60 percent by 1980), and the higher female participation in the workforce, trends that make regular home cooking less likely.

The reintroduction of bread into Yokohama during the late 1850s—to supply the newly opened Western diplomatic and trade posts—was followed in 1869 by the opening of Kimuraya, the first Japanese-owned bakery by Kimura Yasubei. The eponymous store is still in the same location in the very heart of Tokyo (Kimuraya 2010), but the product for which it became famous, *anpan* (bread filled with *an*, a sweetened paste made from *azuki* beans), would not be called bread in Germany or France. Modeled on *manjū*, a steamed wheat (and sometimes rice) flour bun brought from China to Japan in the fourteenth century, this baked (or fried) product is not bread but essentially a kind of sweet bun. Its two original varieties were topped with white sesame seeds (*shirogoma*) and poppy seeds (*keshi*), and Kimuraya still features those two kinds, but as with *manjū*, bakeries across Japan now offer numerous *pan* toppings (including the classic, pickled cherry blossoms) and fillings (ranging from chocolate and custard to curry and pork cutlets).

Soft, white Japanese-type bread is now widely available, as is a multitude of ready-to-eat sandwiches on white bread, and many bakeries now also offer more or less faithful copies of some French, German, and Italian bread varieties. Altogether Japan now produces annually about

1.25 Mt of bread (nearly a third of this being sweet breads), with Yamazaki Baking Company the leading large commercial supplier with nearly 20 percent of the country's market.

Besides bread, buns, and rolls, many other traditional Western baked goods have found solid niches in Japan. Doughnuts are particularly popular (with numerous franchises of Mister Donut, Dunkin' Donut, and Krispy Kreme and with such innovations as "donut burgers"), as are French pastries, cakes (*kēki*), and their Japanese transmutations incorporating *matcha* (powdered green tea) or *kabocha* (winter pumpkin).

The popularity of wheat-based foodstuffs has been reflected in rising per capita intakes but with some interesting fluctuations. Consumption was relatively high in the early 1950s when imports from the United States were compensating for still inadequate rice production. As the rice supply rose, consumption of wheat declined by nearly 20 percent between 1954 and 1957, but in the mid-1960s, it began rising rapidly and peaked at nearly 100 grams per day in 1981. Then came a second stagnation and a slight decline during the 1980s, attributable to higher consumption of animal products, followed by yet another slight rise beginning in the early 1990s, this one due to the greater popularity of wheat-based fast food, bread, and pastries (noodles, buns, bread, doughnuts). In 2000, the per capita consumption of wheat flour was nearly 34.5 kg, compared to about 70 kg in the United States and Germany and 80 kg in France.

Tubers

Potatoes (*jagaimo*) were introduced to Japan during the early encounter with Europeans sometime around the end of the sixteenth century. About the same time, sweet potatoes were brought from China to Ryukyu and established in Satsuma (southernmost Kyūshū) a few decades later (hence their name, *Satsuma imo*). Because of its easy cultivation and fairly good yields (even when the cereal harvest failed), sweet potato became the country's insurance starchy crop and the dominant tuber for more than three centuries, a primacy it retained until the 1960s. Sweet potatoes in Japan have been eaten steamed, baked, dried, candied, and pureed; processed to make starch; and fermented to produce alcohol, vinegar, *shōyu*, and miso. Yam (*yamanoimo*) and taro (*satoimo*) have been the two far more traditional but less productive tubers.

The retreat of Japan's cultivation of potatoes has been in line with a universal dietary trend of a steadily diminishing demand for traditional tubers. Harvests of sweet potatoes rose from about 2.8 Mt in 1900 to 5.5 Mt during the hungry year of 1946 and set the record of 7.2 Mt in 1955; a rapid decline set in afterward, to just over 1 Mt in 2000; the same total was harvested in 2008. In 1900 the sweet potato harvest was more than ten times as large as the potato crop, by 1940 the multiple was down to just over two, by the late 1960s the two harvests became equal, and by the year 2000 the white potato harvest was almost three times as large.

Some traditional tuber preparations are still in demand. Frequent use of sweet potato in tempura, sweet potatoes baked by street vendors in hot pebbles (*ishiyaki imo*) and candied (*daigaku imo*) and some Western potato meals, including potato salad (*potato sarada*) and french fries (*furaido potato*), offered by nearly every fast food chain, became a popular choice (there are even vending machines dispensing hot, but predictably soggy, french fries). But none of this could prevent a long-term decline of tuber consumption, with actual food energy intakes as tubers falling by more than two-thirds between 1950 and 2000, from about 80 to 50 kcal a day and then declining further by more than 20 percent by 2010.

Legumes, Mushrooms, Vegetables, and Fruits

Ancient discoveries of the complementarity of cereal and legume proteins are perhaps the most remarkable examples of a universal and purely empirical solution to a fundamental nutritional problem: the fact that no plant proteins provide a combination of amino acids needed for tissue growth, but that this shortcoming may be overcome by combining lysine-deficient cereals with methionine- and cystine-deficient legumes and hence making it possible to live on vegetarian diets, the norm in all pre-industrial densely populated agricultural societies (Smil 2000). Specific dominant combinations included corn and various beans in the Americas; wheat, rye, barley, and rice, complemented by lentils, beans, and peas in India, the Middle East, and Europe; millets and beans, peanuts, and cowpeas in Africa; and wheat, millets, and rice combined with beans, peanuts, and soybeans in East Asia.

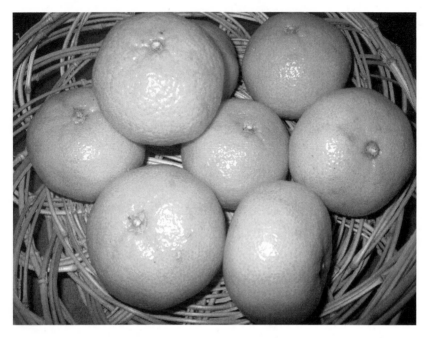

Figure 2.2
An ideal Japanese orange (*mikan*) is easy to peel and has a fine balance of acidity and sweetness. (K. Kobayashi)

Soybeans
The Japanese pattern replicated the southern Chinese combination of rice and soybeans, with other legumes being of secondary importance. Soybeans (*daizu*) came to Japan from China during the eighth century), and it did not take long before their extraordinarily high percentage of protein (between 32 and 40 percent depending on the cultivar, compared to between 20 and 25 percent for most other beans) made them the country's dominant source of this key macronutrient (Watanabe and Kishi 1984). As in China, the contribution of soybeans to the daily diet has been overwhelmingly in the form of processed foods, mainly as *miso* (soy paste), *shōyu* (soy sauce), and tofu (bean curd). Tofu is produced by boiling ground soybeans, with the strained milk traditionally coagulated with *nigari*, seawater-derived magnesium chloride (with some magnesium sulfate). Calcium sulfate, a cheaper coagulant traditionally used in China, was introduced during World War II, and by the late 1950s, almost all Japanese tofu was made with it.

Another important change, the replacement of artisanal tofu production by thousands of small local shops by large-scale industrial processing, began during the 1960s (Shurtleff and Aoyagi 2007). The total number of tofu shops peaked at about 54,000 in 1962; by 2005 fewer than 13,000 were left. Whereas a small shop can process as little as 20 kg of soybeans every day, modern factories process well over 10 tonnes a day, and the yield (of fresh tofu to raw soybeans) increased from less than four in artisanal production to about five for large factories. Per capita consumption in retail weight terms (tofu is 85 percent water) rose from about 6.5 kg a year in 1960 and peaked during the late 1970s at around 16 kg; subsequent decline brought it to about 10 kg a year by the year 2005, with recent consumption being slightly higher (Miura 2009).

Common Japanese tofu (*momen dōfu*) contains about 6 percent protein and is whiter and softer than the yellowish and firmer Chinese *doufu*. Yet another common Japanese tofu, *kinogushi dōfu* (silky tofu), contains more water and less protein but is softer and smoother than *momen dōfu*, since the former is coagulated in the container and undrained, whereas the latter is coagulated before being poured and drained in the container. Tofu is also sold lightly broiled (*yakidōfu*), deep fried in thick (*atsuage*) or thin (*aburaage*) cakes, and freeze-dried (*kōyadōfu*). Soy milk (*tōnyū*) production began in Japan on a small scale in 1954 and increased slowly during the 1960s and 1970s. The drink, now widely available, has never reached the popularity it enjoys in China.

Soy sauce is made by fermenting steamed soybeans and wheat (parched and cracked whole grains) mixed with *Aspergillus oryzae*; the resulting *kōji* is then added to brine and left to mature for at least two years. *Shōyu* (containing about 7 percent protein) became increasingly popular and affordable once its relatively large-scale commercial production began during the early decades of the Tokugawa period (Hayashi and Amano 2005). The two famous makers still in business, Higeta Shōyu and Yamasa, date their beginnings to, respectively, 1616 and 1645. Higeta began by making *tamari,* a by-product of *miso* fermentation made without any wheat, and in 1697 it switched to what became the modern fermentation method (Higeta Shōyu 2009). Beginnings of Kikkoman, now the world's largest soy sauce producer, can be traced to 1661, but its name goes back only to 1964 when it changed from Noda Shōyu, a company established by a merger of family establishments in 1917 (Kikkoman 2010).

Prolonged fermentation of cooked soybeans, a steamed cereal grain inoculated with *Aspergillus oryzae*, salt, and water, produces *miso*: *kome-miso* if rice is used and *mugimiso* if barley is the grain. Brownish-colored red *miso* (*akamiso*) is saltier than the lighter-colored white variety (*shiromiso*). *Miso*, which is 10 to 12 percent protein, is the key ingredient, together with *katsuobushi*-derived stock (*dashi*) and tofu, in miso soup (*misoshiru*), which became a staple during the Kamakura period (1185–1333). The soup was served not only with main meals but also for breakfast, a habit that continues today.

A short fermentation of steamed soybeans inoculated with a bacterium (*Bacillus natto*) rather than with a fungus yields *nattō* (with a protein content of about 16 percent) whose sticky threads are mostly eaten on top of steamed rice and whose peculiar taste is not a great favorite among all Japanese. Young soybean pods are also boiled and the seeds eaten as a vegetable (*edamame*), and the seeds, nearly 20 percent lipids, also yield an excellent cooking oil (containing 85 percent of unsaturated fatty acids). And foodstuffs containing soybeans are marketed as cholesterol-free (iced soy milk tasting like ice cream without any cream, SoyMayo without any egg yolks) or as healthy (Soyjoy bars) choices.

Japan's soybean harvest began to decline decades before rice harvests started to decrease. The annual harvested total was about 450,000 tonnes at the beginning of the twentieth century. It rose to its historic maximum of 550,000 tonnes in 1920 and then began a long period of decline and stagnation as imports from China became available. During the late 1940s, it rapidly recovered from wartime lows, and in 1952 and 1955, it surpassed 500,000 tonnes. Then it resumed its decline and stagnation and ended the century with 235,000 tonnes. Rising postwar imports, first from the United States and, later, smaller imports from Brazil, Argentina, and Canada, have supplied the increasing demand. A brief export embargo on soybeans imposed by the United States on June 27, 1973, which was lifted five days later, did not have any lasting effect on the trade. Since the mid-1970s, imported soybeans have provided around 95 percent of Japan's total consumption, with the United States supplying about 85 percent of all imports between 1956 and 2005 and about three-quarters in recent years (Conlon 2009a).

For many years, there has been an overwhelming chance that such quintessentially Japanese dishes as *yudōfu* (hot tofu), traditionally served in the precincts of Buddhist temples in Kyoto's Higashiyama, or tofu-based *nouvelle cuisine* meals offered by restaurants in Tokyo's Ginza started as seeds harvested in Iowa or Illinois and grown according to Japanese specifications that allow only nongenetically modified varieties and require particular physical and composition properties. These identity-preserved soybeans provide both an assured quality for their users and higher profits for their growers (American Soybean Association 2009). In 2009 nearly half of the total domestic supply of soybeans ended up in processed foodstuffs in high-protein products including tofu, *shōyu*, *miso,* and *nattō* or in soybean oil, and the rest was used (directly or as processing by-products) as animal feed.

The production of green soybeans (*edamame*) has declined by a third from the peak of about 120,000 tonnes a year during the early 1980s, as has the cultivation of the other two most important traditionally grown legumes, kidney beans (*ingenmame*) and red beans (*azuki*). Kidney beans were often just simmered, while small *azuki* seeds have traditionally occupied a more prominent place in the Japanese diet: boiled, ground (in the past manually pounded), and lightly sweetened to make bean paste (*an*, smooth *koshian,* or slightly chunky *tsubuan*) used for filling pastries and *anpan*, or they are added whole to glutinous rice to make a festive *sekihan*. Peak harvests of the two bean crops were reached, respectively, in 1921 and 1930. Other legumes grown more commonly in the past include peas, broad beans, and peanuts. Between the early 1950s and 2010, their consumption fell by 40 percent to only about 70 kcal a day following a virtually worldwide trend. Per capita intakes of both *miso* and *shōyu* have also declined, the former by half between 1960 and 2000 and the latter by about 40 percent (to 8.2 kg).

Mushrooms

Placing mushrooms in the company of legumes is justified on the basis of their high protein content (on a dry-weight basis, fungi contain 30 to 50 percent protein) and relatively high protein quality. Protein digestibility-corrected amino acid scores (PDCAAS) have been the preferred method for evaluating the protein quality of foods because they take into account amino acid requirements for human growth that are adjusted for digestibility of children in the nutritionally demanding age between two and five years of age (Food and Agriculture Association/World Health Organization 1993), Some fungal species have PDCAAS better than those of staple crops that are always significantly deficient in at least one of the eight essential amino acids that adults require. Moreover, the large-scale commercial cultivation of mushrooms uses otherwise worthless agricultural and industrial wastes such as discarded animal bedding, wood chips, sawdust, seed hulls, and banana leaves (Chang and Miles 2004). Some have credited mushroom species with various medicinal effects.

Shiitake (*Lentinus edodes*), a fungus associated with *Castanopsis cuspidata* (Japanese chinquapin, *shii*, of the beech family), has been the most commonly consumed Japanese mushroom. It has been cultivated on hardwood logs for centuries, but large-scale commercial production began during the late 1940s thanks to a new inoculation technique developed by Mori Kisaku in 1943 (Mori 1950; Przybylowicz and Donoghue 1988). The fungus is grown on sterilized wood chips that are embedded into holes drilled in hardwood (mostly oak) logs; incubation lasts up to two years, and fruiting continues for up to six years. At the time of its peak domestic production during the 1970s, Japan's shiitake cultivation employed nearly 200,000 people.

The diminishing availability of suitable hardwood logs and shrinking labor force has resulted in declining domestic cultivation. The fungus is now widely cultivated elsewhere in Asia, and its annual harvest is second only to that of a much more prolific (and much easier to cultivate) species that dominates the Europe and North American markets, *Agaricus bisporus* (*masshurūmu*, the white button mushroom,) whose Japanese cultivation has been also increasing. *Matsutake* (*Tricholoma matsutake*) has been the most highly valued species. As the unrivaled gourmet mushroom of Japan, it sells at exorbitant prices during the fall picking season. Midpriced *maitake* (hen-of-the-woods) is a widely cultivated species. Other commonly cultivated species are *hiratake* (oyster mushroom); *nameko* (*Pholiota nameko*), a small fungus with a gelatinous coating; and *enokitake*.

Japan now imports increasing quantities of mushrooms (fresh, chilled, and dried), with the volume dominated by cultivated shiitake (more than 40,000 tonnes in the year 2000, mostly from China) and value by *mat-*

sutake (annually between 2,000 and 3,000 tonnes) gathered mainly in China, both Koreas, Russia, and Canada. The food balance for the year 2008 shows a total supply of 3.9 kg/capita. Data on actual average consumption of mushrooms from dietary surveys have been available since 1971 when the mean was just 2.8 grams per day (roughly 1 kg per year), while recent means have been as high as 15 grams per day.

Vegetables

As in all other preindustrial societies, vegetables were a critical part of traditional Japanese diet, enlivening the monotony of overwhelmingly cereal-based meals and being the only (or a dominant) source of several essential vitamins and minerals. As elsewhere in East Asia, cabbages, onions, radishes, turnips, carrots, peppers, eggplants, squashes, cucumbers, spinach, and ginger were commonly cultivated species. Perhaps the most distinct feature of traditional Japanese vegetable consumption, and one that persisted during the entire period of the country's dietary transition, has been a widespread pickling of various root and leafy species.

Combinations of pickled vegetables (*tsukemono*) served as a small side dish (*okazu*) with steamed rice is of ancient origin, and the preservation of various leaves, stems, and roots has evolved into a variety of methods yielding unique flavors, textures, and now (with the aid of artificial additives) vivid colors. The simplest way to produce *tsukemono* is to make salt pickles (*shiozuke*), traditionally at home by salting vegetables and weighing them down with stones (*tsukemonoishi*). An ancient method of prolonged pickling of raw or parboiled vegetables in *miso* is still used to produce *misozuke,* as is the perhaps equally old method of using rice bran (*nuka*), to make rice bran pickles (*nukazuke*). All traditional *tsukemono* were heavily salted, but the less salty *asazoke* have become increasingly popular. Even so, consumption of pickled vegetables peaked in 1991, and it is unlikely that a new record will be set.

The Japanese radish (*daikon*) has been perhaps the most commonly pickled plant in Japan. It has been pickled in rice bran (*takuan*), *miso* (*misozuke*), and *kōji* (*bettara-zuke*). Daikon is also eaten fresh, usually finely grated or as thin strands served with *sashimi*. It was quite common to pickle varieties of *Brassica rapa* in salt (*nazuke*). Chinese cabbage (*hakusai*, a white vegetable, Chinese *da bai cai*, also common in hot-pot dishes) joined the *Brassica* species to be pickled after its introduction from China in the Meiji era. Other favorites for pickling include large white turnips (*kabu*), slender cucumbers (*kyūri*), melons (*uri*), eggplants (*nasu*), carrots (*ninjin*), and ginger (*shōga*). Korean *kimchi* (Chinese cabbage–based hot pickle) has recently gained some popularity beyond the country's relatively large population of Korean origin. Western head cabbage (*kyabetsu*) has also become popular, and it is commonly used in salads and soups and to accompany such deep-fried dishes as *korokke* and *tonkatsu*.

Spinach (*hōrensō*) is a favorite among green leafy vegetables, served most often blanched with a dressing using *shōyu* and sesame seeds (*hōrensō no goma ae*). Japanese mustard spinach (*komatsuna*, a leafy variety of *Brassica rapa*) is an ancient cultivar that is rarely found outside Japan and China. Onions (*tamanegi*) go into stews and fries and hot pots, as do green onions (*negi*), but the latter are more often used (thinly sliced and iced) as a condiment. Eggplant (*nasu*) dishes include combinations with *miso* (baked or fried) as well as deep fried (a popular tempura choice), broiled, and simmered preparations. Commonly eaten root vegetables (in soups and hot pots) include turnips (*kabu*) and carrots (*ninjin*). In contrast, Japanese cucumbers (*kyūri*) are always more slender and shorter than the European and American varieties and besides being pickled as *tsukemono* are either eaten raw or prepared in vinegar as *sunomono*. Carrots are also among the favorite for elaborately carved garnishes.

Three introductions from the Americas became very popular: pumpkins, sweet corn, and peppers. Winter squash (*kabocha*) has become a classic cold-season vegetable, boiled or often used in tempura. Corn on the cob (*tōmorokoshi*) is mostly eaten grilled and seasoned, but canned corn often appears in Japanese salads and baked dishes. Favorite Japanese sweet green peppers come in two varieties—one slightly smaller than the Western bell pepper (*piiman*) and the other one so small that looks like a hot pepper (*shishitō*) but is mild. Both are used in tempura, broiled on skewers, or fried with other vegetables.

Several traditional vegetables are still sought after because of their special properties. Rhizomes of lotus (*renkon*) are commonly eaten boiled or pickled and are valued for their crunchy texture and decorative shape, which makes them a favorite addition to boxes full of food for the New Year's celebration. Japanese ginger (*Zingiber mioga*, *myōga*) has a milder taste than common ginger (*Z. officinale*), and it is also a favorite for pickling. The red color of *beni shōga* originally came from pickling it first in salt and vinegar and then adding *akashiso*, red leaves from *Perilla frutescens* of the mint family (also used to color salt-pickled Japanese apricot, *umeboshi*). But the widely available commercial *beni shōga* uses artificial coloring, and *aojiso* (green *shisō*) accompanies sashimi or goes into salads and tempura and is used as a condiment. Ginger is used raw (thinly sliced or grated, particularly with fish dishes) or as pickled *gari*, an indispensable sushi condiment. Fibrous burdock root (*gobō*) is eaten only after shaving and soaking in vinegared water to remove its natural bitterness. Bamboo shoots (*takenoko*) are a typical spring vegetable, eaten boiled, grilled, or as *tempura*.

Finally, a few words about a quintessentially Japanese root vegetable whose name is now well known around the world but it is used to sell an entirely different species. *Wasabi* (*Wasabia japonica*) is usually called Japanese horseradish, but it is not even the same genus as the common horseradish (*Armoracia rusticana*): it is much less harsh and a much more expensive root of the plant that grows wild in clean, shallow streams or is cultivated under cover in wet environment. Because of its high cost (and limited availability in ready-to-use packaging), the real *wasabi* has become only a small segment of what is now a global market in commercial wasabi: its bulk is a powder (paste in squeezable tubes is also available) made from ordinary horseradish, sometimes with added mustard powder; its green color comes from dried powdered *Spirulina* algae or, more commonly, artificial colorants.

Domestic production of vegetables was about 15 percent lower in 2000 than it was in 1975, but the supply changed little due to rising imports. Imports of vegetable were insignificant until the late 1960s, but by they had approached 3 Mt a year. China, Taiwan, Thailand, and Indonesia have been the main suppliers. A combination of falling domestic production and rising imports brought some shifts on the composition of consumed vegetables but few changes to average per capita consumption. The overall weight of vegetables consumed per capita has fluctuated within a narrow range, mostly between 225 and 255 grams per day or between 82 and 93 kg a year, with a slight upward trend during the last two decades of the twentieth century, followed by a slight decline afterward.

Fruits

Traditional domestic fruit production was dominated by *unshū mikan* (*Citrus unshiu*), Asian (or Japanese) pears (*nashi*), persimmons (*kaki*), and *ume* (*Prunus mume*), usually known as Japanese apricot, a species of the genus that includes almonds, apricots, cherries, and plums. *Mikan* is also known as seedless mandarin (*satsuma* after the province from which it was first brought to the United States), but mandarin orange is actually a different species of the same genus (*Citrus reticulata*). *Mikan* is an ancient import from China known for its ease in peeling, usual absence of seeds, and pleasantly sweet taste; most of it is eaten fresh, and the rest is canned, often in syrup. Other citrus species cultivated in Japan include *iyokan* (the second most important cultivar, with harvests amounting to about one-fifth of *mikan*), pomelo (*Citrus grandis, buntan*), and Valencia and navel oranges.

When perfectly ripened, *nashi* combine the best qualities of apples and pears and remain a favorite autumnal choice. *Kaki* (persimmon) is another ancient import from China, and it has been valued as much for its fresh sweet fruit (*amagaki*, as opposed to the famously astringent, mouth-puckering *shibugaki*) as for its preserved (dried and flattened) variety. Unlike their Western counterparts, Japanese apricots are not primarily for eating out of hand but are used either to produce *umeshu* (a sweet liqueur) or the sour, pickled, and salted *umeboshi* that are (colored with *akashiso* leaves) a common accompaniment for rice. By the end of the twentieth century, *mikan* was the only fruit crop with an annual harvest of more than 1 Mt, and apples were second (about 800,00 tonnes), Japanese pears third, and persimmons fourth, ahead of grapes, whose harvest was about twice as large as that of Japanese apricots.

Notably, Japanese statistics classify strawberries, melons, and watermelons as vegetables. The higher intake of a greater variety of fruits has been a common marker of dietary transitions around the world, and the Japanese food choices repeated this trend rather rapidly as domestic production of traditional favorites expanded and imports of both temperate and tropical fruits increased. Between 1950 and 2000, Japan had more than tripled its production of mandarin oranges, nearly doubled its harvest of apples, and more than quintupled its output of Asian pears. Rising incomes brought higher fruit imports: since 1994 more than half of all fruit consumed in Japan has been imported. Apples (imported predominantly in the form of juice) and bananas have been the largest imports, followed by grapefruit, oranges, and pineapples, and by the year 2000, fruit imports had nearly equaled the domestic production.

As a result, by 1980 per capita fruit supply (at about 55 kg a year) was nearly twice the rate in 1960, but by 2000, the rate had pulled back to about 50 kg a year. This means that the country's fruit supply is actually lower than in many Western nations: 80 kg in the United States, almost 100 kg in France, and 110 kg in Germany. But there is a great similarity in the composition of fruit consumption. In recent years, the three most commonly consumed fruits in the United States, Germany, and Japan have been permutations of just three kinds: in the United States, the order is oranges, apples, and bananas; in Germany, apples, bananas, and oranges; and in Japan, apples, oranges, and bananas. France breaks the pattern with oranges, apples, and grapefruit. Per capita fruit consumption doubled between 1950 and 1970, the rate peaked at nearly 195 grams per day (about 70 kg a year) in 1975, then retreated, and since the year 2000 it has fluctuated without any clear trend between 42 and 47 kg a year.

An important segment of Japanese fruit marketing that has seen a great expansion, as well as incorporation of high-quality imported products during the past four decades has been the selling of gift fruits. These specimens, often grown in special ways (also in greenhouses) and selected for their perfect shape, color, and flavor, have traditionally included musk melons, peaches, and grapes, while today's wider repertoire ranges from strawberries to mangoes and from apples to kiwi fruit. Selected fruits are arranged singly or in attractive groupings in decorative packaging, cost often ten times more than ordinary merchandise, and are given as tokens of gratitude, get-well gestures, or presents to important clients.

Seafood

Japan's seafood is a close equivalent of the French or Italian umbrella terms *fruits de mer* and *frutti di mare*, which include crustaceans (lobsters, crabs, prawns, shrimp), mollusks (muscles, oysters, clams, scallops), cephalopods (squid, octopus, cuttlefish), and fish (from tiny smelt and bottom flatfishes to eels and large tunas), but no other country in the

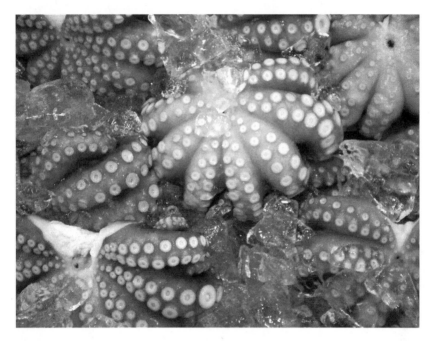

Figure 2.3
Besides scores of fish species, the Japanese diet also contains many marine inver-
tebrates. This picture shows cooked common octopus at Tokyo's Tsukiji market.
(V. Smil)

world consumes such a variety of species belonging to all of these categories. Moreover, no other country matches Japan in consuming as much
plant food (so many different varieties of seaweeds) from the sea.

Seaweeds

Various species of seaweeds have been traditionally harvested, processed
(usually dried), and eaten in other Asian countries (above all, in China
and Korea, as well as in Southeast Asia), in parts of Europe (notably
Irish moss in Ireland and winged kelp in Ireland, Scotland, and Brittany)
and North America (dulse in eastern Canada) and in Hawaii and New
Zealand—but in none of those countries have they become such an
essential part of common diets as in Japan (McHugh 2003). Even so,
their contribution to overall energy and protein supply is negligible, but
they are valued above all for their high mineral and vitamin content, as
well as for their medicinal properties.

Because it serves as a wrap for the now ubiquitous *makizushi*, *nori* (processed sheets of purple laver, algal species of *Porphyra* genus growing in the intertidal zone) is easily the most recognizable Japanese seaweed outside Japan (Miyashita 2004). Cultivated on nets suspended near the surface in coastal waters (and exposed to air for a few hours a day), the algae start yielding multiple harvests in just seven weeks after seeding, and their output now leads Japan's maricultural production, ahead of oysters and yellowtails. Traditional hand preparation of *nori* has been entirely superseded by mechanical processing to make standard 19- by 21-centimeter dry sheets that weigh 3 grams and are used to wrap sushi and *onigiri* (normally after toasting, producing *yaki nori*), added to soups and noodle dishes and boiled down in *shōyu*.

Toasted *nori* can be also flavored and eaten on its own as *ajitsuke nori*. The characteristic taste of *nori* is due to its relatively high levels of several amino acids, and the alga has a high protein content (30 to 50 percent), as well as high concentrations of vitamins A and C and some components of vitamin B. *Aonori* (green laver) is a minor cultivated seaweed that comes from an entirely different algal genera (*Monostroma* and *Enteromorpha*) and is used for flavoring various foods in dried and powdered form. Genus *Laminaria* (*konbu*, Japanese kelp), a large-leafed brownish plant from cold coastal waters with a naturally very high content of glutamate, is the second most important group of seaweed harvested for food. All of it used to come from the natural kelp beds of Hokkaidō and northern Honshū, but about a third of the annual consumption is now cultivated. The alga has much lower shares of protein and vitamins than *nori*, but it contains iron and iodine. Most notably, it is an essential ingredient in preparing Japan's all-purpose stock (*dashi*); it is also eaten boiled with other vegetables in soup or in *shōyu*.

Deep green, thin-stranded *wakame* is sold both salt-pickled and dried, and it is a standard ingredient in *misoshiru* and in many salads. *Hijiki* is a brown sea grass that turns black when boiled before drying and is added to various foods because of its high fiber and mineral content (above all, calcium and magnesium, but it also has a relatively high presence of arsenic). Perhaps its most popular use is in *hijiki mame*, combined with soybeans, *shōyu*, and sugar. *Tengusa* is a red alga harvested for its high content of a polysaccharide that is extracted to produce agar (*kanten*), a gelatinous substance used as a growth medium in laboratory cultivation of bacteria and fungi, food processing, and the preparation of visually appealing desserts. *Anmitsu* is agar dissolved in water or fruit juices and served with sweet bean paste or with fruits, while semitranslucent *yōkan* (agar combined with *an* and sugar and sometimes flavored with *matcha* or other plant-based pastes) is served during tea ceremonies.

Cultivation of *nori* goes back to 1600, and for centuries it relied on collecting natural spores on bundles of twigs, and later on nets, placed in estuaries (Tamura 1966). Reliable large-scale cultivation became possible only after Kathleen Drew's discovery of the life cycle of *Porphyra* made artificial seeding techniques possible (Drew 1949). As with many other foodstuffs, Japan has become a growing importer of seaweeds, mostly from China (mainly *wakame*) and South Korea (mainly *hijiki*), with Chile, Brazil, and Tonga being minor suppliers. Since 2000, seaweed imports have been around a third of the total supply. Slightly more than a fifth of all available species are used as feedstocks for industrial processing (mainly extraction of agar), and exports have been less than 3 percent of domestic production. Seaweed consumption (in fresh weight terms) rose from 3 grams per day in 1950 to nearly 7 grams per day by 1970 and then has fluctuated mostly between 5 and 6 grams per day.

Fish and Marine Invertebrates

There are major maritime nations where this category would not warrant a great deal of coverage in comparison to other animal foods. Germany's annual per capita supply of fish and seafood (all rates in terms of live weight) has been always less than 15 kg, both the U.S. and the British rates have been recently just above 20 kg, and the Canadian rate, despite the nation's three oceans, has been no higher than 25 kg, or just slightly below the Italian mean. Among the major Western economies, only the French average around 30 kg. In contrast, in 2008 Japan's seafood harvest amounted to just over 5 Mt, and net imports boosted the overall supply to about 9.4 Mt, or nearly 75 kg/capita. Among major economies, only South Korea (with an average per capita seafood supply about 15 percent lower than in Japan) is in a similar category. Another revealing way to look at Japanese seafood consumption is to note that the nation's average per capita supply of crustaceans, cephalopods, and mollusks is larger than the total per capita seafood supply in the United States or United Kingdom.

After subtracting nonhuman consumption (mostly as feed in the country's extensive coastal mariculture), recent average per capita food supply rate was about 55 kg a year, or approximately 150 grams per day. As expected, seafood consumption entails a relatively great degree of waste: fish heads, guts, bones, fins, and invertebrate shells account for at least 40 to 45 percent of live weight. In 2008 the overall yield for Japan's seafood was 56 percent, leaving 4 Mt (about 31.5 kg a year) for actual consumption. Nutritional surveys show per capita consumption rising from just 55 grams per day in 1946 to the peak of 98 grams per day in 1997, followed by a decline to 86 grams per day by 2008 (Ministry of Agriculture, Forestry and Fisheries 2008b).

Japanese statistics distinguish three categories of fish catches—pelagic, offshore, and coastal—but the historical data series of catches by species are not strictly comparable due to changes in the survey coverage and the reassignment of some major species (skipjack and tuna). With these caveats in mind, it is interesting to note that the share of coastal catches fell from about 75 percent during the 1930s to just 20 percent by 1975—but then it rose again to just over 30 percent by the year 2000, while the share of offshore catches has remained relatively stable, mostly between 40 and 45 percent. Official statistics show the total fish and marine invertebrate landings rising from nearly 1.6 Mt in 1900 to the prewar peak of about 4.3 Mt in 1936 and the postwar landings rose from just 1.8 Mt in 1945 to the peak weight of 10.75 Mt in 1986 before falling by more than 50 percent (table 2.2; graph 2.2a).

Japanese mariculture was expanding fairly steadily between the late 1940s and the late 1980s before it reached a plateau between 1.2 and 1.3 Mt a year (total including seaweeds, invertebrates, and fish), while inland water fisheries and freshwater aquaculture more than doubled between the early 1950s and the late 1970s. By 2005, however, their contribution (at just 100,000 tonnes per year) was no higher than it was a half-century before. In aggregate, the net domestic supply of seafood doubled between 1960 and 1980 and peaked in 1988 at 13.5 Mt. By the century's end, it declined by 20 percent, and in the year 2008, it was down to 9.4 Mt as Japanese catches and mariculture were once again slightly ahead of imports. As a result of these trends, Japan's seafood catch is now only the world's fifth largest (behind China, Peru, the United States, and Indonesia and ahead of India and Thailand), and in 2007 its aquacultural output

Table 2.2
Aquatic production, imports and supply, 1900–2008

Year	Total production (catch and aquaculture) (Mt)	Net imports[a] Mt)	Supply[b] (Mt)	Average annual supply[c] (kg/capita)	Tuna catches[d] (10^3 tonnes)	Tuna imports[d] (10^3 tonnes)
1900	1.6	—	1.6	36	15	—
1925	2.9	—	2.9	49	33	—
1935	4.0	—	4.0	57	68	—
1950	3.4	—	3.4	40	59	—
1965	6.5	—	6.5	65	430	10
1975	9.9	—	10.0	89	311	115
1990	10.3	2.7	13.0	105	293	257
2000	5.7	5.6	10.8	85	286	362
2008	5.0	4.2	9.4	74	230	228

a. Denotes quantities of less than 0.1 Mt.
b. Totals take into account annual changes in stocks and include food for direct consumption and processing as well as the aquatic species used as feed.
c. All values are rounded to the nearest kilogram.
d. Includes albacore, bigeye, bluefin, skipjack, and yellowfin tuna.

ranked ninth (China leads, India is second, and Japan comes behind Chile and Norway). In 2007 Japan also lost its status of the world's largest importer of seafood as the United States pulled slightly ahead.

Traditional coastal Japanese fishing was dominated by catches of just a few species. During some prewar years, sardines (including anchovy) accounted for more than half of the total weight, followed by herring, cod, and mackerel, with the top three species accounting for about 70 percent of the total catch. As the Japanese fishing fleet extended its area of routine operation, the composition of its catch has changed, and its variety has tended to increase. In 1950 sardines were still the top catch (about 25 percent of the total), but the top three species (sardines, mackerels, and herring) made up only about 40 percent of the total catch. By 1975 the order changed again, with cod at nearly 30 percent, followed by mackerels and sardines, and the top three species added up to just over 50 percent of the total catch. By 2000, sardines were again at the top of a greatly reduced overall catch, and the top three species (anchovy, skipjack, and cod) brought less than 40 percent. Five years later, the share of the top three catches remained roughly the same, but the order now

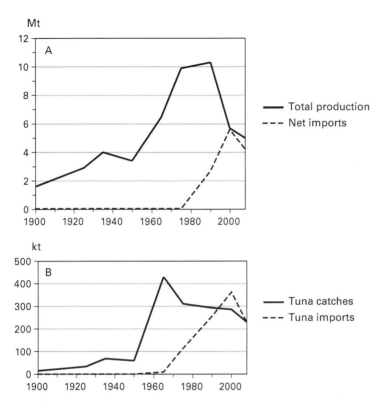

Graph 2.2
Production and imports of whole aquatic species (A) and tuna (B) in Japan,
1900–2008.

was mackerel, skipjack, and anchovy (Ministry of Agriculture, Forestry,
and Fisheries 2007).

Collapse of sardine (*ma-iwashi*) stocks has been the most dramatic
development, from nearly 4 Mt a year harvested in the mid-1980s to less
than 30,000 tonnes by 2005, but catches of mackerel (*ma-saba*), Japanese anchovy (*katakuchi-iwashi*), and skipjack (*katsuo*) remain high,
with mackerel accounting for nearly 20 percent of the total catch. Other
important species are Pacific saury (*sanma*), jack mackerel (*aji*), ara-
besque greenling (*hokke*), salmon (*sake*), and Alaska pollock (*suketōdara*).

No other category of fish has been more emblematic of Japan's seafood
consumption than various tunas. Japan has the world's largest tuna-
fishing industry, and it is also the leading importer and consumer of these
large, sleek fish species, all of which have been under increased fishing

pressure and some of whose stocks have been perilously reduced by over-fishing (Bergin and Haward 1996; World Wildlife Fund 2010). Fortunately, that is not the case with *katsuo*, the most commonly caught tuna (its recent Japanese catches have fluctuated between 300,000 and 400,000 tonnes annually) whose Pacific stocks appear to be high and in no danger of overfishing. The fish is eaten in a variety of ways—raw (both as *sashimi* and sushi), seared (*katsuo no tataki*), even fermented (*katsuo no shiokara*)—but in terms of constant presence in Japanese cuisine, no other seafood product is as important as *katsuobushi* (Miyashita 2000).

The traditional way of making this unique product begins by boiling the flesh, deboning it, and smoking it for hours to days in order to reduce its water content; this is followed by drying and curing. *Katsuo* chunks are then placed in chambers rife with *Aspergillus glaucus* (also with *A. ochraceus*) whose growth reduces the moisture further and imparts a distinct (*umami*) taste and is stopped after about two weeks by drying. Repeated sequence of molding and drying produces chunks of meat as hard as wood that must be shaved before use. This used to be done with a small wooden plane (*kezuriki*) just before cooking, but poor households in the past and busy users now prefer a shaved product, either in bulk packages or in small portions suitable for a single meal. Large shavings (*kezuribushi*) are used to make *dashi*, the basic stock in Japanese soups, as well as in liquids used for simmering, dressing, and dipping. A combination of inosinate from *katsuobushi* and glutamate from *konbu* produces a pronounced *umami*. Smaller shavings (*itokezuri* or *usukezuri*) are used as a topping for boiled vegetables and tofu and as a stuffing in *onigiri*.

For most of the past fifty years, yellowfin (*kihada*) and bigeye (*mebachi*) have had very similar catches, mostly between 100,000 and 130,000 tonnes a year, and both of them have now declined to less than 100,000 tonnes. As a result, yellowfin imports (of mostly frozen fish) have recently surpassed the domestic landings, and as Japan's catch of *mebachi* declined, its imports (fresh fish mainly from Indonesia and Palau, frozen fish mainly from Taiwan and China) have increased to more than 60 percent of the total supply, which has been averaging about 250,000 tonnes a year (Sonu 2007). *Mebachi* is used mostly for sashimi and sushi, and so is yellowfin, whose meat is softer, blander, and much less fatty (and hence less expensive) than that of bluefin tunas.

Albacore (*binnaga*) is now the fourth most important tuna species landed in Japan. Its catches have fluctuated considerably during the past fifty years, but they have not shown any clearly declining trend, and the country remains the leading albacore producer, ahead of Taiwan and Spain (Sonu 2006). As a result, albacore imports have also fluctuated widely, but they have accounted for less than 10 percent of the overall market. Most of the albacore catch is canned, with only a small part sold as steak or as sashimi and sushi. But it is the rarest of all tunas, bluefin (*maguro* or better yet *hon maguro*, true tuna), with three species: *kuro maguro*, Pacific bluefin (*T. orientalis*), *taiseiyō kuro maguro*, northern bluefin (*T. thynnus*), and *minami maguro*, southern bluefin (*T. maccoyii*)— whose consumption has become the iconic embodiment of Japan's fish culture (Hori 1992, 1996).

Maguro was not a highly prized fish during the early Edo period, and it became popular only with the diffusion of *edomaezushi* during the nineteenth century when *akami*, the less oily meat of the red inner muscles, became a favorite sushi *dane* (topping). Eventually preferences shifted, and now the most desirable cuts for sashimi and sushi come from the sides just below the midline (*chūtoro*) and the fatty belly (*ōtoro*). Pacific bluefin has been traditionally caught in waters east, southeast, and south of Japan. No nationwide statistics for tuna catches are available prior to 1951, but a reconstruction of fish landings in major ports on Hokkaidō, Honshū, and Kyūshū (Muto et al. 2009) indicates that annual catches from coastal fisheries remained mostly between 5,000 and 8,000 tonnes until the mid-1920s. Subsequent introduction of drift nets pushed the annual catches above 30,000 tonnes by the mid-1930s. Postwar recovery and extension of long-distance fisheries brought new record bluefin catches, with the peak of just over 70,000 tonnes in 1961.

Subsequent decline from the late 1980s has brought the annual levels (few exceptional years aside) to less than 20,000 tonnes (table 2.2; graph 2.2b). But this decline in Japanese catches has been accompanied by rising consumption as the country's bluefin imports rose from less than 5,000 tonnes per year during the mid-1980s to a record of over 52,000 tonnes in 2006 (Sonu 2008), and the share of the imported bluefin in the total supply rose from less than 20 percent in 1985 to nearly 75 percent in 2007. Bluefin exports to Japan have been a lucrative business.

Most fresh bluefin (gilled and gutted, with the tail off) comes from Mexico and Australia. Australia and Croatia have become by far the largest suppliers of frozen fish, with their deliveries now coming overwhelmingly from farmed fish: young tunas are captured by purse seines and then moved to large offshore cages where they are fed sardines, mackerel, herring, and processed feeds for three to six months. Spawning the fish in captivity has been a challenge, however, and although progress has been made, wild stocks remain highly endangered (Masuma et al. 2008; Australian Seafood Cooperative Research Center 2009).

Before leaving this brief survey of important fish species consumed in Japan, it is necessary to mention the puffers, or blowfish (*fugu*). These species have highly poisonous skin, ovaries, and liver, but their thinly sliced translucent meat (or a soup, *fugu chiri*) can be eaten safely when the fish is eviscerated and sliced by an expert. Nevertheless, every year there are reports of some adventurous gourmands suffering mild tetrodotoxin poisoning and, though rarely, death. Recent catches of *fugu* have fluctuated rather widely, between 7,000 and 11,000 tonnes a year, while Japanese *fugu* mariculture produces about 5,000 tonnes a year.

Marine invertebrates are an important part of Japan's overall seafood harvest, with various species of squids (*ika*, with common squid, *Todarodes pacificus*, dominant) making up nearly 10 percent of all marine catches, while shellfish, mostly scallops (*hotategai*), contributed about 4 percent. Shrimp (*ebi*), lobster (*ise ebi*), and crab (*kani*) catches have been declining, and these seafoods now come mostly from imports. In contrast, mariculture is dominated by just three species: in 2000, more than half of marine fish culture were yellowtails (*inada* or *hamachi*), and all but a small fraction of shellfish aquaculture was split between scallops and oysters (*kaki*).

Given the quantity and the variety of seafood consumed in Japan, it is hardly surprising that fish, shellfish, and mollusks have been served in many ways, from live animals and raw tissue to highly processed foodstuffs. Eating raw seafood (as well as raw freshwater fish and invertebrates) is an ancient tradition whose reach has been greatly extended by modern food preservation and transportation techniques that have made freshly harvested (or deep-frozen) foodstuffs widely available. Mostly thinly (but sometimes fairly thickly) sliced sashimi, appealingly presented with shredded *daikon* and *shiso* garnish, and various kinds of sushi are the two quintessential Japanese ways of consuming raw seafood, and they have become increasingly accepted in other parts of Asia as well as in Europe and the Americas.

The original form of this compound food (*narezushi*) was made by months-long fermentation of salted fish in rice (Yoshino 1986). Any fish and many crustaceans and mollusks can be used to prepare sashimi, but *maguro, saba, hamachi, ebi, ika,* and *tako* are traditional favorites, with farmed salmon now often used. *Shōyu* is always used for dipping sashimi, and wasabi may or may not be present. Smaller slices of raw seafood pressed onto an oblong rounded bit of vinegar-flavored rice (*sushi meshi* or *sumeshi*) form *nigirizushi* or *edomaezushi* because its fish came from the waters of the Edo Bay when sushi became a popular food choice in the Tokugawa capital during the last half-century of *shōgun* rule (Uchida 1989). And some 150 years later, during the closing decades of the twentieth century, sushi became Japan's most successful culinary export.

There is also pressed sushi (*oshizushi*) formed inside a wooden mold with seafood pressed on top: various kinds of seafood scattered on a generous serving of rice (*chirashizushi*) and *temakizushi* with fish morsels inside (and almost spilling out) of a rather loosely hand-rolled rice-filled cone made of *nori*. None of these three arrangements is now as popular as many varieties of *makizushi* (originally served along with *nigiriszuhi*): tightly rolled assemblies of seafood (and other ingredients), rice, and *nori*. Traditionally these rolls used to be made as small *nori*-wrapped cylinders about 2 centimeters across (*hosomaki*) or as wider *futomaki* (fat rolls, about 5 centimeters across). Classical *hosomaki* contained only a single filling, with cucumber (*kappamaki*), tuna (*tekkamaki*), and *kanpyō* (seasoned gourd strips) rolls being the great favorites. In contrast, a *futomaki* usually has two or three complementary (taste- and color-wise) fillings. The wrapping is not limited to *nori*: sushi wrapped in a thin omelet (*chakin-zushi*) and in fried tofu (*inarizushi*) have been popular since the Edo era. Inside-out rolls (*uramaki*) are a modern American addition to the genre, as are various colorful rolls wrapped in seafood or thin slices of vegetables and fruits.

Grilled fish (*yakizakana*) is a common dish, prepared without marinating or marinated in *miso, shōyu,* or special sauces; salt-grilling (*shioyaki*) is a traditional way of fish preparation, with *sanma* a favorite species. Grilling is also used to prepare a favorite summer dish, freshwater eel (*unagi*) that is then glazed and grilled over charcoal (*unagi no kabayaki*). Seafood is also stewed (*nizakana*), sautéed (*munieru*), fried, and deep-fried, with deep frying being used to prepare one of Japan's signature dishes, batter-dipped seafood *tempura*, originally a Portuguese import of the sixteenth century that now features *ebi* and *ika* as the most common seafood choices. Boiled seafood is prepared as either *suimono* (clear broth) or *nabemono* (one-pot dishes). A substantial amount of Japanese cooked seafood is eaten cold as a part of the ubiquitous lunch box (*bentō*), where it accompanies rice and pickles. As already noted, there is no tradition of oven baking. Steaming, a favorite way of cooking fish in China and Southeast Asia, is also a traditional way of food preparation in Japan, but the Japanese *mushimono* usually contains a mixture of ingredients (including seafood) rather than an entire fish as in China.

Pureed fish meat, or fish pastes (*gyoniku neri seihin*, for those familiar with the French cuisine best imagined as firmer versions of *quenelles de poisson*), are made of *surimi*, ground white meat of several fish species, with Alaskan pollock, Pacific croaker, whiting, and cod the most commonly used varieties. Their ground meat is combined with salt, starch or flour, egg whites, sugar, and seasonings, and then it is shaped and steamed. It is sold in tubular forms (*chikuwa*, originally molded around bamboo tubes), in small semicylindrical loaves presented on rectangular pieces of wood (*kamaboko*), in little square cushions (*hanpen*), or as fried pieces (*satsuma age*). As with all other seafood products, *surimi* imports (mainly from the United States, Thailand, China, and India) have been increasing.

Smoking, a traditional form of preservation in many European countries (salmon in northern Europe, mackerel and herring in the Netherlands and Germany), has been relatively unimportant in Japan. Instead, salting and drying have been traditionally adopted for preserving fish as well as aquatic invertebrates. Even in the early twentieth century, salted fish was only an occasional treat in inland villages. But fresh fish has not entirely replaced preserved fish products. Salted (and often dried) fish products are much less salty than they were in the past and are now chosen because of their unique tastes rather than because of their long shelf lives.

Whales

The last seafood item we describe might be also included in the next section on meat. Whale meat (from animals killed near Japan's coasts) was eaten throughout the country's recorded history because the recurrent bans on killing and eating animals did not apply to sea mammals, and whales (*kujira*) were classed as *isana*, a large fish (Shiba 1986). Consumption of whale meat (*geiniku*, raw or salted), internal organs, and blubber became more common during the Edo period when whale skin soup became a favorite. Modern whaling with harpoon guns on steamship bows began in 1899, and long-distance expeditions to the North Pacific and the Antarctic Ocean started in 1934. By 1925 Japanese whalers had killed about 1,600 animals (mostly sperm whales), and by 1939 the annual total rose to about 9,800. Whale meat supply reached about 10,000 tonnes by 1925 and 45,000 tonnes in 1939, with per capita availability of, respectively, about 170 grams and 630 grams a year (Ishida 2009).

Postwar restoration of whaling assumed an instant importance in the hungry nation. In 1946 whale meat supplied nearly half of the country's scarce animal protein, in 1947 it was the only meat served in school lunches. It remained the leading source of animal protein during the late 1950s and the early 1960s. Large-scale hunts for whales were dominated by factory ships (their numbers peaked at eighty-six in 1962) operating in the Antarctic waters (Ishida 2009); whaling in northern waters and near the country's coast was much less important. Whale meat supply peaked in 1962 at nearly 2.4 kg/capita (mostly from fin, sperm, and sei whales). The total number of killed whales peaked in 1965 with nearly 26,000 animals, and the industry remained fairly strong until the mid-1970s, when about 13,000 whales were killed every year. It then declined rapidly, with just over 5,000 whales killed in 1980.

In 1982 the International Whaling Commission (IWC, established in 1946 to regulate the hunt and conserve whale stocks) responded to a widespread opposition to whale killing and imposed a moratorium on commercial whaling starting in 1986 (Kalland and Moeran 1992). But whale meat did not disappear from Japanese stores. Although the country observes the ban on commercial fishing, it continues a small-scale hunt of whales (mostly minke, as well as a few sei and sperm whales) with the private, nonprofit (but government-supported) Institute of Cetacean

Research in charge of the hunt and Kyōdo Senpaku owning the vessels and doing the meat processing and marketing. This activity has been producing annually between 1,000 and 2,000 tonnes of whale meat, and a few hundred tonnes come from coastal whaling for smaller species and also from some dolphins (Ishihara and Yoshii 2003; Institute of Cetacean Research 2010). Norway and Iceland have been the only other countries defying the moratorium.

Whale meat continues to be sold in stores, and whale dishes are served in restaurants that specialize in them (Ohnishi 1995; Nippon Research Center 2006). Red whale meat (*akaniku*) is most often eaten as sashimi, as is *unesu*, the cut of meat and fat from the animal's ventral (lower jaw and belly) region that is also used to make whale "bacon." It is also boiled with *shōyu* and used to make burgers and meatballs and during the 1950s and 1960s was turned into sausages. Yet culturally based and sometimes emotional arguments about the merits and importance of whaling (appealing to Japan's traditions and cultural uniqueness) are becoming increasingly irrelevant, as even the small amount of whale meat that has been available in Japan, Iceland, and Norway fails to find eager consumers. In more recent times, the annual supply reached its highest levels in 2005–2006 at about 5,600 tonnes, but a significant share of this meat has remained unsold and was kept in cold storage (Greenpeace 2009).

As whale meat prices dropped in 2005, *geiniku* began to be used once again (two decades after it had been replaced by chicken or pork) as burgers and meatballs to schoolchildren in some parts of Japan, but not surprisingly, some of these meals were found to contain very high levels of methyl mercury. Attempts to revive whale meat consumption will most likely continue, but Kyōdo Senpaku estimated that all whale meat sold in Japan in 2008 as a by-product of ICR activities amounted to just 50 grams per capita, or just three or four slices of sashimi, an entirely negligible quantity of animal protein and hardly worth international attention.

There are virtually no prospects for any return to substantial whale meat consumption. Japan's three largest fishing companies that were the former leaders of commercial whaling (Maruha Nichiro, Nihon Suisan, and Kyokuyō) have stated that they would not resume the hunt even if the IWC lifted its ban, and public opinion polls show that more than 60 percent of Japanese have not eaten whale meat for a long time (for many older people, this would mean since they were children or teenagers, because the meat was served at school lunches until the 1970s), about 20 percent have never tasted it, and a large majority of people think that the future demand for whale meat will remain at the same low levels as now or that it will drop even more (Nippon Research Center 2006).

Meat, Eggs, and Dairy Products

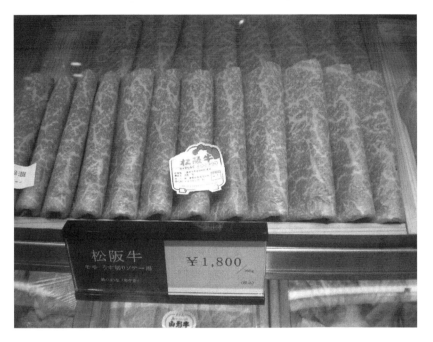

Figure 2.4
The high price of Matsuzaka beef—1 kg costs more than $200—is due to its high fat-to-meat ratio. (V. Smil)

A combination of environmental factors (most of the Japanese islands are forested mountains, lack extensive pastures outside Hokkaidō, and have limited arable land) and religious proscriptions (Buddhist bans on eating domesticated animals) made animal breeding a negligible component of medieval and early modern Japanese farming. The meat of wild animals was eaten (with varying frequency) even during the centuries when the edicts proscribed its consumption, but average consumption of pork, beef, and eggs remained very low and there was a virtual absence of dairy foods. While most of the preindustrial European countries also had low, or even very low, per capita rates of meat consumption, milk and cheese were more commonly available. Meat and dairy segments of Japan's dietary modernization had to start almost from zero, and in the latter case the transition did not begin until after the end of World War II, which makes the current relatively high per capita intakes of red meat and poultry and widespread consumption of milk and processed dairy foodstuffs even more remarkable.

Red Meat and Poultry

Although Japanese traditions regarding meat eating and its proscriptions can be divided into several distinct periods, the boundaries between those periods are fuzzy. In the pre-Buddhist Japan, wild animals were hunted, and deer and pigs were eaten. Buddhist *ahimsa*, defined by Vyasa's commentary on *Yoga Sutras* as "the absence of injuriousness (*anabhidroha*) toward all living things (*sarvabhuta*) in all respects (*sarvatha*) and for all times (*sarvada*)," is one of the cardinal tenets of the faith (Chappel 1993). Adherence to Buddhist beliefs introduced from Korea around the middle of the sixth century was the principal reason for the imperially dictated prohibition of meat eating, including domesticated mammals, as well as poultry and monkeys in 675 C.E. (Ishige 2001; Watanabe 2008). Imperial ordinances forbidding the killing of animals and eating of meat were proclaimed repeatedly during the Asuka and Nara periods between 676 and 781. Moreover, there were various *shintō* taboos on the eating of cattle, horses, and, particularly, fowl, which were seen as announcers of dawn rather than a source of food, and these taboos were generally respected until the fifteenth century (Ishige 2000).

Centuries after the original ban, further restrictions were put in place during the Kamakura period (1192–1333), requiring fasts following any meat consumption to make the practice widely unacceptable. Meat eating was reintroduced locally and regionally by Christian missionaries during the second half of the sixteenth century and despite renewed bans on killing and eating animals in 1687, the meat of wild animals (above all boars, deer, and hares) was eaten not only by hunters in mountain villages but in some cities by the second half of the eighteenth century.

During the late Tokugawa period, meat was more widely available, but per capita consumption remained minuscule as meat was still seen as a marginal, medicinal food preferably reserved for those experiencing sickness and weakness. In 1869 the government set up Gyūba kaisha (Beef and Pork Company), and in 1871, it changed the official attitude regarding meat eating by declaring meat to be important for good health. In 1872 it was announced that the Meiji emperor was eating meat regularly, meat became a part of army rations, and even Buddhist monks were permitted to eat it (Ishige 2001; Watanabe 2008). The reaction to this change (both approval and consternation) was strong, but before the end of 1870s, more than 500 butcher shops were open in the capital (Harada 1989).

Nevertheless, domestic meat production remained small, and with only token meat imports, the overall per capita supply remained minuscule. In 1900 the annual meat supply (in terms of carcass weight) prorated to only about 800 grams per capita (mostly beef), by 1925 it was about 1.7 kg (roughly 50 percent beef, 40 percent pork, and 10 percent horse meat), and in 1939 it was almost exactly 2 kg/capita, that is, still only about 5 grams per day, or no more than 3 grams a day in terms of edible meat and fat. Obviously much as throughout the Southeast Asia and in Mediterranean Europe, regular meat eating was not a part of typical daily Japanese prewar diet, and the meat supply remained very low during the first two postwar decades as well. In 1950 the carcass weight of domestically produced meat was no higher than during the late 1920s.

By 1960 domestic meat supply (with imports accounting for less than 7 percent) reached 6.5 kg. Rapid increases of domestic output began during the mid-1960s, with the total doubling between 1965 and 1974 and then growing by another 50 percent by 1984. Concurrently, imports kept rising, from 10 percent of the total supply in 1965 to 20 percent by 1985. The annual per capita availability of meat nearly tripled between 1965 and 1985, from 12 kg to 35 kg. Domestic output peaked in 1987, then declined to 3 Mt by 1996, and it has been holding around that level ever since. In contrast, meat imports rose to 2.7 Mt by the year 2000 and then stabilized close to that level (table 2.3; graph 2.3a). In terms of carcass weight, the average meat supply was nearly 45 kg/ capita by the year 2000, or about 29 kg in actually edible portions, nearly a sixfold increase since 1960.

There have been also some significant shifts in the composition of the Japanese meat supply. Horse meat (*baniku*, also called, because of its color, *sakura niku*) remained a nonnegligible contributor (on the order

Table 2.3
Meat production imports and supply, 1900–2008

Year	Production (Mt)	Imports[a] (Mt)	Supply[b] (Mt)	Per capita supply[c] (kg/year)	Average annual consumption[d] (kg/capita)		
					Chicken	Pork	Beef
1900	0.03	—	0.03	0.7	—	—	0.5
1925	0.08	—	0.08	1.3	—	0.7	0.6
1935	0.09	—	0.09	1.3	—	0.7	0.6
1950	0.12	—	0.12	1.4	0.1	0.7	0.6
1965	1.1	—	1.1	11	2.1	4.1	2.3
1975	2.2	0.4	2.6	23	3.6	10.3	6.7
1990	3.5	1.3	4.8	39	13.5	15.3	8.4
2000	3.0	2.8	5.7	45	15.4	17.6	10.1
2008	3.1	2.5	5.6	44	15.2	18.6	9.0

a. Denotes quantities of less than 0.1 Mt.
b. Totals take into account annual changes in stocks.
c. Starting in 1965, all values are rounded to the nearest kilogram.
d. Supplies not shown include horse, mutton, lamb, goat, and poultry other than chicken.

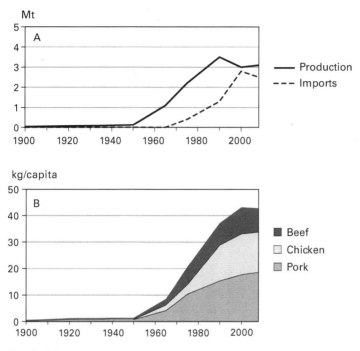

Graph 2.3
Animal meat production and import (A) and per capita annual consumption (B),
1900–2008.

of 10 percent) until the late 1950s. Its domestic production peaked in
1962 at about 25,000 tonnes; it then declined rapidly and since the mid-
1970s has fluctuated between about 4,000 and 7,000 tonnes a year. Most
of the horse meat now consumed in Japan (about 3 percent of all meat)
is imported, with Argentina, Brazil, and Canada being the leading exporters. The meat is eaten raw (*basashi*) or cooked in a hot pot (*sakura nabe*),
and Kumamoto prefecture (western Kyūshū) has been the center of both
horse meat production and consumption. As horse meat began its retreat
during the 1960s, consumption of chicken (quite negligible during the
1950s) nearly quintupled: in 1960 it accounted for only 15 percent of
all meat, by 1980 it surpassed a third of the total, and that share was
little changed by the year 2000. In per capita terms, that meant a rise
from 0.8 kg a year in 1960 to 10.2 kg a year in 2000; at that level, its
consumption was about a third higher than that of beef and nearly as
high as that of pork.

Chicken (*tori niku*) has become a common choice for both Japanese and Western-style meals and their assorted combinations and fusions. Among the most popular choices are chicken *yakitori, teriyaki,* fried chicken (*karaage*), chicken one-pot (*mizutaki*), chicken and egg rice bowl (*oyakodon*), chicken *tempura,* and chicken curry. Less common is the Japanese equivalent of chicken risotto (*tori zōsui*) and fried or simmered chicken meatballs (*tsukune*). Chicken is readily available in its various deep-fried forms at nearly 1,000 KFC (*Kentakkī furaido chikin*) restaurants and other fast food outlets (KFC Japan 2010).

Per capita pork and beef supply were roughly equal in 1960, before the country's meat popularity took off, but by 1970, pork consumption was 2.5 times and by 1980 2.7 times higher (graph 2.3b). Subsequent liberalization of beef imports reversed the trend, and by the year 2000, the ratio of pork to beef was about 1.4. Actual per capita pork intakes rose from 1.1 kg in 1960 to 11.7 kg in 2008 (table 2.3). This means that pork remains Japan's most popular meat, with chicken about 10 percent lower. Pork (*buta niku*) can be found in simmered dishes (*buta kakuni*), curries (*pork karē*) and soups (*tonjiru*), hot pot (*buta-shabu*), rice bowls (*katsudon*), and ground or minced in meatballs.

Pork can also be found in a variety of Chinese-style or Western-style dishes: stir-fried with vegetables, as filling in fried or steamed dumplings (popular *gyōza* and *shūmai*) and spring rolls (*harumaki*), and as deep-fried *tonkatsu*. *Tonkatsu* is Japan's popular variant of breaded European pork cutlet. It was introduced during the Meiji era and has acquired a status of Japanese food (*washoku*) by being served with rice and *tonjiru* and cut up into pieces to be eaten with chopsticks. *Katsudon* is an embodiment of the fusion of the European and Japanese cuisine: a bowl of rice topped with *tonkatsu*, onion, and egg seasoned with *shōyu*-based sauce.

Beef consumption has lagged the supply of pork and chicken not because of a significantly lower demand (based on traditional or taste preferences) but because beef was not available in sufficient amounts for decades and this relative scarcity drove and sustained its high prices. In 1960 beef was no more expensive, and sometimes even slightly cheaper, than pork and chicken. By 1980 domestic production of pork was nearly ten times the level of 1960, and for chicken the rise was nearly elevenfold. In contrast, between 1960 and 1980, Japan's beef production, increasingly expensive and unable to approach the productivity gains of other meat-producing sectors, only tripled while imports remained highly restricted. As a result, by 1980 beef cost about three times as much as chicken and more than two and a half times as much as pork.

The history of Japanese meat imports in general, and beef in particular, is a convoluted sequence of domestic restrictions, quotas, levies and tariffs, and foreign pressures to lower trade barriers and open the Japanese market (the major milestones are described in detail by Longworth 1983 and Conlon 2009b). In relative terms, overall meat imports more than doubled between 1960 and 1968 to about 15 percent of the total supply, but it took twenty years to reach 25 percent. Then came a big spurt: meat imports were a third of the total supply by 1992 and came very close to 50 percent by the year 2000, with beef accounting for nearly half of this rapid rise. In per capita terms, Japan's beef supply rose from only about 2 kg in 1960 to almost 8 kg in 2000 (table 2.3). Not surprisingly, this was only about a quarter of the average U.S. rate and roughly a third of the French or Italian supply but only about 25 percent less than the per capita beef availability in Germany.

The most expensive kinds of domestically produced beef (*gyū niku*) come from crosses of traditional black-coated, small-stature *Tajima-ushi* breeds of *wagyū* (Japanese cattle used for centuries as draft animals) and European animals, and they have achieved cult status in both Japan and abroad. Kōbe beef from Hyogo prefecture—produced by feeding heifers in pens for up to three years, regularly massaging the animals, and giving them beer to drink during the summer—is so highly marbled (20–25 percent of marbled fat, compared to 6–8 percent for USDA prime beef) that its most expensive cuts look more white than red and are sold for more than $500/kg. Matsuzaka beef (from Mie prefecture) is even more expensive and has an extremely high fat-to-meat ratio: these cows are also fed beer in summer and massaged with *shōchū* (Japanese liquor).

The quintessentially Japanese use of beef is in the form of thin slices for *sukiyaki* and *shabushabu* meals or in rice bowls (*gyūdon*). Westernization of the Japanese diet has brought more frequent use of beef in grilled (*yakiniku*) and curried dishes and in beef and potato stew (*niku jaga*). Since the 1970s ground beef has been almost as widely available in Japan as in any Western country that has been invaded by American hamburger chains. McDonald's hamburgers (*Makudonarudo hanbāgā*) came to Japan in 1971, and the country now has the second largest number of the restaurants — about 3,600 compared to nearly 13,000 in the United States and about 1,100 each in Canada, the United Kingdom, and Germany (McDonald's Japan 2010). Burger King and Wendy's also compete in Japan, together with domestic hamburger chains led by MOS Burger (since 1972), Freshness Burger, First Kitchen, Lotteria, and Sasebo Burger. While restaurants selling hamburgers are ubiquitous, steak houses, which are usually very expensive, are uncommon, as is home cooking of large pieces of beef, be it by roasting, grilling, or barbecuing.

Eggs

Proscription of animal foods in Japan's medieval diet meant that egg consumption began to make its first small inroads only after the fifteenth century, but it remained an insignificant source of high-quality protein until after 1950. In contrast to the previously negligible egg consumption, an average Japanese now consumes more eggs in a year than an average American or a citizen of the European Union. Unlike in China and in the countries of Southeast Asia, the Japanese diet has never included duck eggs, and small speckled quail eggs (*uzura no tamago*, eaten raw and in soups and *nabemono* dishes) have been much less important than hen eggs (*tamago*). These are also consumed raw, in soups, and in *nabemono*, as well as in such signature Japanese dishes as chicken and egg on rice (*oyako don*) and sweet omelets (prepared with *dashi, shōyu* and *mirin*) that are eaten alone or often added to *bentō* boxes and used as a common *sushidane*, often fastened with a thin strip of *nori*.

Egg production data begin in 1906 when the output was just about 35,000 tonnes or 750 grams per capita, an equivalent of fifteen small eggs per year, but this official figure is likely an underestimate. By the late 1930s, per capita supply rose to one egg per week, the bottom was reached in 1946 with fewer than two eggs per year, prewar highs were regained only by the mid-1950s, and by the early 1990s, the supply reached a plateau at about 20 kg, an equivalent of a large egg per day per capita. Japan's egg supply has been thus about 30 percent higher than in major Western economies: in France, Germany, and the United States, it averages around 15 kg per capita. Recent imports have been less than 5 percent of the total supply.

Dairy Foods

Japan's remarkable renewed embrace of meat eating has been, along with declining intakes of staple carbohydrates and increasing consumption of a greater variety of fruits, part of a universal pattern of dietary transition. In contrast, Japan's post–World War II adoption of dairy products as part of an everyday diet has been truly exceptional. The embrace of dairy food represented a notable shift in a country that did not practice milking domesticated animals for hundreds of years and whose population has a high prevalence of lactose intolerance or lactase deficiency (Suarez and Savaiano 1997). Milking is well documented in Japan of the Heian period (794–1185); afterward it became a rarity, and in 1868, at the time of the Meiji restoration, there were no more than 500 Brahman milch cows in Japan, descendants of a Dutch gift of three heads to the *shōgun* in 1727 (Watanabe 2008).

Lactose intolerance is a genetic trait due to low levels, or a near absence, of lactase, the enzyme responsible for digesting milk sugar, after early childhood. Infants, with the exception of a very small share of genetically disadvantaged (or prematurely born) babies, well tolerate lactose (a sugar made up of glucose and galactose) in maternal milk, but their intestinal concentration of lactase declines substantially around the age of five in populations that have no history of milking domestic animals and have not been consuming milk and dairy products throughout their lives. In contrast, a mutation of a dominant genetic trait that has evolved during more than 10,000 years in populations that have been drinking large quantities of milk throughout their recent evolution as pastoralists or sedentary farmers has maintained adequate lactase activity in parts of Europe, the Middle East, India, and Africa (Simoons 1978; Kozlov et al. 1998). In contrast, lactase deficiency reaches its highest frequency, with rates of at least 70 percent to virtually 100 percent, among the traditionally nonmilking populations of sub-Saharan Africa and East Asia, including Japan.

When the absence, or a low level, of lactase prevents lactose absorption, the sugar's bacterial fermentation in small intestines produces gases (which often cause abdominal discomfort and cramping) and fatty acids (which can lead to diarrhea, and some people even vomit after drinking milk). And yet these realities have not prevented an impressive increase in Japan's consumption of dairy products. Three reasons explain why. First, in most adults with lactose intolerance, lactase synthesis is not completely turned off, so they can consume milk without discomfort as long as they drink only a small amount at one time. Not surprisingly,

Yoshida et al. (1975) found a milk intolerance of only about 19 percent in Japanese adults with intakes of up to 200 milliliters, or slightly less than a cup of milk—and regular drinking of just a cup of milk a day would add up to about 80 liters a year, fairly high consumption.

Second, such fermented dairy products as buttermilk, sour cream, and yogurt have nearly as much lactose as whole milk, but the bacterial enzymes present in these foodstuffs act as substitutes for the absent endogenous lactase and make digestion easier. Third, unripe cheeses contain only a small fraction of the initial lactose (less than 30 percent for such unripe varieties as cottage cheese and ricotta), and all fully ripened varieties have virtually no lactose left (Hui 1993), so the limit on their consumption is a matter of taste and expense rather than one of digestive discomfort. The Japanese experience is a perfect illustration of adopting a food group that has been not only entirely absent from the traditional diet, but remained quite insignificant during the early decades of modernization and whose importance rose rapidly only from the 1950s. Neither the high prevalence of lactase deficiency nor the ancient cultural bias has been able to prevent this remarkable dietary innovation.

Japan's historical statistics trace raw milk output since 1906, when it prorated to a negligible per capita availability of less than 2 milliliters per day. Subsequently Japan's milk production grew relatively slowly, but almost without interruption, to reach about 392,000 tonnes (or 5.4 liters per capita) in 1941; by 1946 it collapsed to less than 150,000 tonnes. The rapid growth of output began in 1950 and continued, though at a diminishing rate, until the 1980s. During the 1950s, nationwide output more than quintupled as the annual per capita supply rose to 20 liters as milk was served by the national school lunch program.

Takahashi (1984) concluded that the unprecedented growth in the average height of children during the fifteen years between 1960 and 1975 (almost equal to the gain of the thirty-year periods between 1900 and 1930 and 1930 to 1960), as well as the disappearance of a previously uneven spatial pattern of childhood growth and obvious urban–rural discrepancy, has been due mainly to increased consumption of milk, although higher consumption of meat, egg, and fish protein and better preventive health measures also contributed to this trend.

By 1970 domestic milk output averaged about 45 liters per capita. By 1990, it reached a plateau around 66 liters, and by 2010 it had declined to below 65 liters. Production is heavily concentrated on Hokkaidō, and the three largest dairy companies (*Meiji Nyūgyō, Morinaga Nyūgyō,* and *Yukijirushi Nyūgyō*) command nearly 40 percent of Japan's total milk market. Between 55 and 57 percent of Japan's domestic milk output is sold as fluid milk, and the rest goes for processing into dairy products (condensed and evaporated milk, skim milk powder, butter, cheese, ice cream, and yogurt). Imports of dairy products began with dry U.S. milk right after the war. Imports of butter and cheese increased slowly during the 1970s and then took off during the late 1980s. When converted to a fluid-milk basis, they have been above 2 Mt ever since (Obara, Dyck, and Stout 2005; Obara 2009).

By the year 2000, the supply of dairy products (converted to fluid milk basis) reached nearly 95 kg/capita, and fluid milk was about 40 percent of that total. The National Milk Promotion Association's 2002 survey of more than 4,000 individuals found that only 11 percent of respondents did not drink any milk, 15 percent did not eat any yogurt, and 19 percent did not consume any cheese (Watanabe and Suzuki 2006). Modal drinking volume was about 200 milliliters a day, and a third of all respondents ate yogurt one to four days a week; cheese was consumed much less frequently—one or two days a week by 20 percent of respondents and just two or three days a month by a quarter of the sample.

By the year 2000 the share of fluid milk as the total of all dairy consumption (compared on fluid milk basis) reached about 40 percent, close to the level prevailing in most Western nations and near the threshold of saturation for milk drinking. The validity of this threshold was confirmed by a statistical analysis of perceptions and attitudes regarding milk drinking and consumption of yogurt and cheeses: its results indicated that very little can be done to increase milk drinking (Watanabe and Suzuki 2006). Subsequent developments confirmed this conclusion as milk drinking stagnated and then began to decline, with average consumption per household falling from 94 liters in 2006 to 86 liters in 2008 (Obara 2009). Average consumption of butter, cheese, and yogurt also declined, and the trend intensified in 2009, with milk drinking falling by about 10 percent. Per capita supply of dairy foodstuffs (calculated from food balance sheets) was about 34 liters of fluid milk, about 0.5 kg of butter, and 2.2 kg of cheese; no data are available for yogurt (Ministry of Agriculture, Forestry and Fisheries 2008a).

Despite the recent decline in the demand for dairy products, their total annual per capita supply expressed in mass terms on a fluid milk basis is well above the total weight of rice or seafood. In 2008, at about 86 kg, it was about 32 percent higher than the supply of milled rice (65 kg) and more than 50 percent higher than the availability of all seafood (56 kg). Obviously the comparison is different in food energy terms as milk is mostly water: 3,500 Kcal/kg of digestible energy in rice, 2,000 Kcal/kg in seafood, and 650 Kcal/kg in milk. Rice is still the single largest source of available food energy, but dairy products have come very close to the seafood, and in terms of its frequent consumption, milk has become a staple food in Japan: four out of five Japanese are aware of its high nutritional quality, and it is now consumed regularly in more than 80 percent of all households (Campo and Beghin 2005) and by about 90 percent of all Japanese.

At the same time, dairy products in Japan are, and will almost certainly remain, a secondary staple, unlikely ever to attain the importance they hold in Western European, Australian, or North American diets. Japan's annual averages of about 35 liters of milk, less than 1 kg of butter, and about 2 kg of cheese are still far below the EU means of about 80 liters of fluid milk, nearly 5 kg of butter, and 17 kg of cheese. But comparisons with other traditionally nondairy Asian countries are more appropriate, and they show Japan well ahead of South Korea and China, whose annual milk supply rates in 2007 were, respectively, about 45 and 30 liters per capita.

More remarkably, Japan's supply of dairy products is not very different from that of India, where the cow is a sacred animal and dairy products—milk (*doodh*), butter (*makhan*, or in its clarified form as *ghee*), buttermilk (*chaach, mattha*), cheese (*paneer*), yogurt (*dahi*, or in its churned and iced form as a drink, *lassi*)—have been the only important animal foods in an otherwise purely or overwhelmingly traditional vegetarian diet. India's fluid milk supply reached about 95 liters per capita in 2007, just marginally ahead of the Japanese rate. But because of India's lower per capita food availability, the share of food energy derived from dairy products is slightly higher than in Japan.

Japan's annual food consumption surveys indicate that per capita intakes of all dairy products rose roughly tenfold between 1946 and 1960 (to about 33 grams per day), more than doubled during the 1970s, and has been above 100 grams per day ever since. Consumption peaked at 170 grams in 2001, and the subsequent decline brought them to between 125 and 135 grams per day, or nearly 50 kg a year. Recent years have seen some relatively high declines of both fluid milk and butter consumption. Because many people among the aging and generally more health-conscious population choose soy milk instead of cow milk, it is unlikely that even in the long run, today's per capita levels of fluid milk (or yogurt and cheese) consumption will increase significantly, and it is also unlikely that any possible increases in cheese and yogurt intakes could create a rising demand.

Other Foodstuffs and Beverages

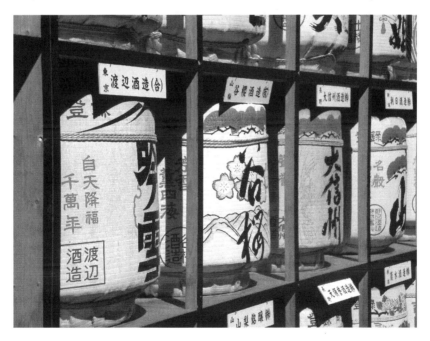

Figure 2.5
Saké is Japan's leading indigenous alcoholic beverage. Drumlike empty *saké* containers are often displayed at temple grounds, here at Hie jinja in Tokyo. (V. Smil)

Before closing this review of changing supply and consumption of major food groups, we look at three additional classes of dietary transformations: the changing consumption of fats and oils (a shift from traditional Japanese diets that were exceedingly low in any lipids), sweeteners in Japanese diet (again, a shift from traditional diets that used no or only token amounts of, sweeteners to consumption of pastries, ice cream, and sweetened drinks), and the changing habits of drinking, a rapid postwar shift that has led from the dominance of tea and *saké* to widespread embrace of coffee, carbonated soft drinks, and a wide selection of Western alcoholic beverages ranging from wine to distilled spirits and liqueurs.

Fats and Oils

Animal fats (butter, lard, tallow) and oils derived by pressing seeds of annual plants (corn, soybeans, rapeseed, peanuts, sunflowers, sesame) and nuts (walnut, coconut) have been essential ingredients in traditional Western cuisines: their use results in higher food energy density and a greater palatability of many dishes, and they are indispensable components of meaty (as well as vegetarian) sauces, stews, pan fries, and roasts. They go into baked products ranging from simple crackers to ornate cakes, oils dress salads, and solid fats have been favorite bread spreads. Preindustrial consumption of fats and oils was widely limited due to low incomes, and their increased consumption has been one of the most obvious markers of the Western transition to richer diets, with an interesting post-1960 shift in overall lipid composition as the use of butter (and even more so of lard) declined and as polyunsaturated (corn, rapeseed, soybean) and monounsaturated (olive) oils rose in popularity.

In contrast to the Western norm—as well as in contrast to the most common Chinese cooking method, stir-frying, which needs at least a little bit of plant oil or animal fat to coat small pieces of meat, vegetables, or tofu that are quickly cooked over high heat—traditional Japanese cooking used almost no added fat. Virtually all of Japan's common meal preparations—*nimono* (simmered foods), *nabemono* (single-pot dishes), *mushimono* (steamed food), *yakimono* (grilled foods), *aemono* (cooked salads), *sunomono* (vinegared salads), and *suimono* and *shirumono* (soups)—could do entirely without any added lipids. In premodern Japan, only the richest among the urban elites could afford to deep-fry foods (*agemono*) frequently, and the popularity of deep frying expanded significantly only after World War II.

Consequently it is not surprising that the traditional intake of lipids (overwhelmingly of plant origin) was so low that until the late 1950s, they supplied less food energy on an average day than vegetables did. Subsequently, lipid intakes tripled by the mid-1980 (to about 150 kcal a day), but during the 1990s, they began falling and are now once again only at about 90 kcal a day, the level first reached during the mid-1960s. Butter remains relatively unimportant, and the lipid supply is dominated by cooking oils. Rapeseed oil has been Japan's most important plant lipid since the mid-1980s, followed by soybean oil and palm oil. Corn oil comes fourth, ahead of rice bran oil, which is still more important than olive oil.

A small share of these plant oils is produced from domestically grown soybeans and rice bran; the rest is pressed from imported seeds (above all, from rapeseed and soybeans) or purchased abroad (palm oil). Soybeans come mostly from the United States, rapeseed from Canada (Australia is a secondary supplier), olive oil from Italy and Spain, and palm oil from Malaysia (Food and Agriculture Organization 2011a). The total domestic supply of plant oils more than quintupled between 1960 and 2000, and dietary surveys show consumption rising from just 2 grams per day during the 1950s to the peak of 15 to 17 grams per day (roughly 5.5–6.2 kg a year) until 2000 and then a significant decline to less than 10 grams a day. At only about 3.5 kg a year, Japan's per capita consumption of plant oils remains far below the Western average of around 25 kg a year in the United States and mostly between 15 and 20 kg a year in the EU.

Sugar

Modern dietary transitions have always brought higher intakes of sugar, but in Japan's case, the increase has remained relatively low. As in nearly all other preindustrial societies, Tokugawa Japan had a negligible (and mostly medicinal) consumption, and, as in China, sugar was never used to sweeten tea. Domestic sugarcane cultivation began during the early eighteenth century, but nearly two centuries later, during the Meiji era, sugar was still used merely as an accent sweetener to flavor some simmered vegetables and sukiyaki, and to make *wagashi*—traditional Japanese confections using glutinous rice, azuki beans, chestnuts, yams, and agars—eaten when drinking *matcha* (Yamamoto 2007). Makers of *higashi*, the best-quality *wagashi* made from fine raw rice flour, have been using *wasanbon*, a superfine cane sugar that has been produced for 200 years by traditional artisanal methods in Tokushima and Kagawa in Shikoku.

Both sugarcane and sugar beet cultivation began to expand during the last decades of the Meiji era, with cane production roughly doubling between 1900 and 1914 and then staying close or just above 1 Mt per year until 1939. But most of Japan's prewar sugar consumption came from Taiwan (under Japanese control between 1895 and 1945). By 1910 Taiwanese sugar provided about 75 percent of the total supply, and by 1935 its share was about 90 percent (Mitsubishi Economic Research Bureau 1936). As a result, per capita supply of sugar rose from only about 1 kilogram in 1900 to about 16 kg by 1939. Wartime sugarcane cultivation then virtually collapsed, and the postwar domestic sugar production has been dominated by sugar beets whose harvests have been above 1 Mt a year since 1949. In 2000 the combined production of beets and cane produced nearly 800,000 tonnes of raw sugar, but twice that amount was imported.

Even so, Japan's total sugar supply has remained very low when compared to both other affluent nations and some low-income countries where sugar is used to sweeten tea (International Sugar Organization 2009; World Health Organization 2009). Japan's supply of sweeteners had doubled between the late 1950s and 1980, leveled off afterward, and declined by 10 to 15 percent beginning in the 1990s. Annual per capita supply of sugar rose rapidly from almost nothing in 1946 to 5 kg in 1950, and it peaked at nearly 30 kg in 1973. This rise was followed by about two decades of declining demand to only 19 kg/ capita in the year 2000.

In contrast, in the year 2000, the EU per capita sugar supply averaged about 37 kg, that in the United States 32 kg, and Brazil 58 kg (World Health Organization 2009). Although the traditional very low-sugar diet is gone, Japan has not embraced excessive sugar consumption either: it still derives less food energy from sugar than any other affluent country. Japanese dietary surveys do not have an aggregate category of sugar and other sweeteners (as the FAO's food balance sheets do) but offer two relevant groupings: "sugar and preserves" and "confectionery and sweets." Obviously not all food energy in the processed foodstuffs included in these two categories comes from added sugar. In lightly sweetened *wagashi*, it comes from starches and in Western-type chocolates from lipids (cocoa butter). But whatever their actual sugar content is, overall consumption of these products has remained stable since the early 1960s, at just over 100 kcal a day.

Confectionary production, dominated by chocolates, has been about 350,000 tonnes per year, with Lotte and Meiji Seika being the largest domestic makers. Imported chocolates are widely available, and some foreign brands have accommodated Japanese taste preferences to a hard-to-believe degree. Kit Kat chocolate bars (*kitto katto*), introduced by Rowntree in the United Kingdom in 1935 and now made by Nestlé, are made in scores of varieties, many of them available only in specific regions of the country, an exclusivity that makes a perfect choice for inexpensive *omiyage* (gifts brought from travels). These choices, with a postcard-like address panel on the back so they can be conveniently mailed, include such unusual chocolate flavors as green tea from Kyoto, *shōyu* from Tokyo, and *wasabi* from Shizuoka (Kit Kat 2010). Another Japanese chocolate-related custom is the Valentine's Day custom of women giving sweets to men. Japanese *depātō* (department stores) cash in on this demand by offering limited editions of expensive chocolates.

Tea, Coffee, and Soft Drinks

Green tea and *saké* are inseparable from the foreign image of the Japanese diet, but unlike European wines and beers (with their ancient history of widespread and frequent consumption), those two quintessentially Japanese beverages do not have a very long history of common, everyday use. A stern Tokugawa ordinance issued to villages in 1649 made it clear that the peasants "must not buy tea or *saké* to drink, nor must their wives," and it was not until the late eighteenth and the early nineteenth centuries when slowly rising incomes made these two beverages common, first in the largest cities and later in the better-off rural areas.

Japanese tea—*cha*, or *ocha*, or *nihoncha* as opposed to *kōcha*, the fermented teas traditionally consumed in the West—is yet another import from China (no later than early ninth century) that has been transformed into a quintessential ingredient of not only of the Japanese diet but also of the country's cultural identity (Varley and Kumakura 1989; Kyōto Kokuritsu Hakubutsukan 2002; Ohki 2009). Japanese tea stands apart from the final product of the world's other major tea-producing cultures because of the minimal processing of the harvested leaves of *Camellia sinensis*, a medium-sized, densely leaved perennial bush. Unlike the semifermented teas of China (oolong) and fully fermented and often flavored and even smoked teas in India, Sri Lanka, and southwest China, Japanese green tea (*ryokucha*) is unfermented. Although the production of numerous varieties of Chinese green teas begins with pan-frying the harvested leaves in order to stop their oxidation (fermentation), in Japan the same goal is achieved by steaming the leaves before they are dried.

Basic categorization of *cha* runs from the most commonly drunk coarse-leaved, even twiggy *bancha* (and its roasted variety, *hōjicha*, both brewed with boiling water) to good-quality teas (*sencha*) containing young leaves and steeped only briefly in water no hotter than 80°C and to the most select pickings of *gyokuro* grown in shade and brewed with water at just 50°C. Powdered *matcha*, made famous by its use in the Japanese tea ceremony, is also produced from high-quality leaves. Addition of roasted brown rice to ordinary teas produces *genmaicha*, a nutty-tasting brew. Two other less common varieties, and at the opposite ends of the quality spectrum, are *kabusecha*, a high-quality *sencha* whose leaves are shaded before the harvest, and *kukicha*, a tea made from stems, stalks, and twigs of the tea plant. An expanding segment of the Japanese market offers black oolongs with high levels of polyphenols that are approved by the Ministry of Health, Labour and Welfare for weight control; other teas target, even less credibly, "beauty-conscious" women.

Japanese tea production rose from about 28,000 tonnes in 1900 to 62,000 tonnes by 1941, and the postwar output peaked in 1978 at about 105,000 tonnes per year. Subsequent decline has kept the output below 100,000 tonnes a year. Japanese tea imports were negligible (at just a few percent of the total supply) until the late 1960s, but since the early 1990s, they have been at more than 35 percent of domestic tea consumption. More than two-thirds of the imports are green and semifermented teas from China; most of the rest are fermented teas from Sri Lanka, India, Indonesia, and Kenya. Conversely, Japan has benefited from the rising popularity of green tea abroad: its tea exports rose from just over 300 tonnes in 1990 to nearly 1,800 tonnes in 2007.

The Japanese habit of tea drinking remains strong, but for the past fifty years, it has been under pressure from a new and vigorous rival: coffee. Although Tokyo's first coffeehouse opened in 1899, coffee remained uncommon until the 1960s. Since that time, Japan has not only become the world's third largest importer of coffee (behind the United States and Germany), but it has been consuming more coffee than tea by weight and value since 1975 (Euromonitor International 2009). The Japanese coffee market has some notable peculiarities: instant coffee brands (led by Nestlé) have always dominated the overall sales; canned coffee and coffee in PET bottles (both widely available from vending machines) are important segments of the total market; females (especially those between twenty-five and forty years of age) have been the main consumers of freshly brewed coffee; and international chains (Starbucks, Doutor, Tully's) provide intense competition for the largest domestic providers of fresh coffee: UCC Ueshima, Key Coffee, and Art Coffee.

Coffee drinking began to make its first significant (urban) inroads only during the late 1960s: by 1975 the annual per capita supply surpassed 1 kg (and it equaled the weight of tea), and it was 3.5 kg by the year 2000. This amount of beans would be enough for 500 to 550 servings of European coffee (depending on the size of the servings and its strength), or about 10 cups a week. For comparison, 1.1 kg of tea consumed annually per capita in the same year would yield, with 2.25 grams needed for a cup, 500 servings, putting Japanese per capita tea and coffee drinking roughly on par in terms of consumed liquid volume.

In reality, large volumes of these beverages are not consumed in dainty china cups but in ready-to-drink, canned, or bottled form. Unlike in other affluent countries, tea drinks are the largest segment of Japan's enormous soft drink market (with about 6 billion liters produced in the year 2008), followed by carbonated drinks and coffee drinks (each at about 3 billion liters in 2008); next in order are mineral water and sports drinks (both with rising consumption since 2000) and fruit drinks (falling consumption), all close to or just above 2 billion liters in 2008. Smaller categories (all well below 1 billion liters per year) include lactic drinks, vegetable drinks, and soy milk (Japan Soft Drink Association 2009). Among the leading brands, Georgia Coffee (a Coca-Cola brand introduced in 1994) came first in 2005, followed by Itōen's Ōi ocha green teas, Aquarius sports tonics, and various colas.

The extent of Japan's soft drink market is indicated by the fact that some 300 new products are introduced every year (most of them never succeed), and that in addition to large food stores and small convenience outlets, Japanese can buy these drinks from about 3 million vending machines. Overall per capita consumption of these drinks now amounts to more than one standard can a day. The Japanese soft drink market is also known for such offerings as Placenta 10000 (a drink containing an extract from pig placenta) and Kona Deep Deep-Sea Drinking Water, desalinated water drawn from the deep ocean (Business Wire 2006; Keferl 2008).

Black vinegar (*kurozu*) drinks (containing 5 percent acetic acid, more than standard vinegars) have been other recent favorites sold for their purported beauty-enhancing qualities. And there are many more unusual beverage choices, including (perhaps most famously and most ineptly named) Pocari Sweat (a sports drink that now ranks among the top ten in overall sales) and Deepresso coffee. By volume, about 60 percent of these drinks are now sold in plastic bottles, with metal cans a distant second, followed by paper containers and aluminum cans. But as with many other aspects of Japan's dietary transition, there are clear signs of demand saturation for fresh coffee as well as for coffee, tea, and fruit drinks and tomato juice: since 2005, per capita consumption has been stagnating or declining for all of these categories. This trend is related to the aging of the population and the world's fiercest competition among beverages as market shares shift without an overall increase in sales.

Alcoholic Beverages

Competition between tea and coffee has had its counterpart in the contest between *saké* and *shōchū*, the only two alcoholic beverages produced in Japan until the Meiji restoration, and Western alcoholic beverages, starting with beer brewing during the closing decades of the nineteenth century and after World War II also including rising imports, and domestic production, of wine and distillates. Production of *saké* begins with highly milled rice, and the degree of milling determines the drink's two major categories: for *ginjōshu*, rice containing less than 60 percent of the whole grain is used, and for *honjōzō*, milling goes down to only 70 percent (Kondo 1984; Gauntner 2002). *Junmaishu* (much like the beer brewed according to the German Reinheitsgebot of 1516 that can contain only malted barley, hops, yeast, and spring water) is made of only milled rice, water, and *kōji* (more than 15 percent of milled rice on a weight basis). Sugar or pure alcohol is added to other *saké* varieties, and *futsūshu*, ordinary *saké* that accounts for more than three-quarters of all sales, also contains added organic acids.

Steamed rice is inoculated with *kōji* (rice infected with *Aspergillus oryzae*, the mold that is also used in producing *shōyu* and *miso*) and yeast, and it undergoes parallel saccharification (conversion of starches to sugar) and alcoholic fermentation (conversion of sugar to ethanol). Pressing, pasteurization, filtration, dilution with water, and aging may precede the final bottling, and the presence or absence of these processes determines other *saké* classifications: undiluted *genshu* has 17 to 20 percent of alcohol; light filtering produces milky-looking *nigorizake*; sherry-like *koshu* is a result of two to five years of aging; aging in casks yields woody-tasting *taruzake*; and there is also unpasteurized *namazake* (Japan Sake Brewers Association 2010). Traditional *saké* was much thicker and sweeter than the dry and light varieties that have dominated the market since the 1960s and whose alcohol content of 14 to 16 percent is comparable to the most alcoholic natural red wines or Spanish sherry.

Shinohara's (1967) reconstructions make it possible to trace average annual *saké* consumption since 1876 when it was 17 liters per capita, or nearly 3.5 liters of ethanol per capita, a very high consumption for such a traditional, low-income society. For comparison, U.S. consumption in 1870 was nearly 7 liters of ethanol per person of drinking age (U.S. Bureau of the Census 1975). By 1900 Japan's *saké* consumption had risen slightly to 20.2 liters, and subsequent decline brought it to 12.2 liters in 1935. That level of per capita consumption was not reached again until the late 1960s, and after a temporary plateau at around 12 liters per capita, it began to decline to just above 4 liters by 2005. Japan's whisky production had an even steeper rise and fall, reflecting the pre-1990 boom and the post-1990 economic weakness. Domestic output doubled between 1965 and 1970 and then grew by another 70 percent by 1975, but by 2005 it was no higher than in the early 1960s.

In contrast, the popularity of *shōchū* has been increasing. *Shōchū* is Japan's traditional distilled spirit that can be made from any grains and tubers, in Japan most commonly from barley (*mugijōchū*), rice (*komejōchū*), or sweet potatoes (*imojōchū*) and whose legal alcohol content should be no more than 36 percent (in practice, it is anywhere between 20 and 40 percent, with an average of 25 percent). Multiply distilled *kōrui* has virtually no odor, but *otsurui* is made with a single distillation and hence carries a very distinct smell of its starchy feedstock, be it rice or brown sugar. Per capita consumption of *shōchū* had declined from about 3 liters during the late 1950s to just over 1.5 liters two decades later but by 1990 it was close to 5 liters per year. In 2000 the production of *shōchū* surpassed that of *saké*, and by 2005 the mean was just over 8 liters per year, with all major brewers (Asahi, Kirin, Suntory) introducing new brands.

Commercial beer brewing was introduced during the 1870s, and by 1886 domestic production (greatly beholden to the imported German expertise) began to surpass imports (Francks 2009). Subsequent consolidation of the industry and emergence of a few dominant producers pushed the output from about 2.5 million liters in 1890 to about 312 million liters by 1939 (Fuess 2003). Average annual consumption rose from less than 100 milliliters per capita in 1890 (when most Japanese never tasted the drink) to about 2.5 liters per capita by the mid-1930s. Beer brewing had virtually collapsed during the war, but afterward it kept expanding in step with Japan's economic growth, and by the year 2000 it reached about 53 liters year.

That is very similar to annual beer drinking in Sweden and Norway, roughly half the rate in Austria and Australia, and a third of the rate in the global record holder, the Czech Republic. But even at that moderate level, beer has become Japan's most important alcoholic beverage: its production surpassed *saké* output more than half a century ago, and by the year 2000, the volume of beer output was more than nine times larger, and even when adjusted for the lower alcohol content (5 percent versus 15 percent of ethanol) it was still more than three times as large. Big players on the Japanese beer market (Asahi, Kirin, Sapporo, Suntory, Orion) keep introducing new varieties, and they have developed low-malt beer (*happōshu*) in order to escape higher taxes; it now claims nearly a third of all domestic sales.

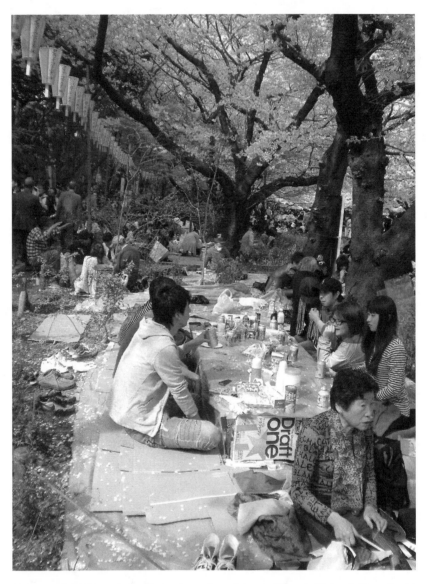

Eating and drinking under flowering *sakura* (pictured here in Tokyo's Ueno Park) exemplifies the continuity and change of Japanese foodways: a traditional pastime modernized by drinking canned soft drinks and beer and eating Western snack foods. (V. Smil)

3

Food Consumption: Continuity and Change

Chapter 2 traced the important components of Japan's diet, from rice to seaweeds, and the long-term changes in supply and per capita consumption. In this chapter we quantify Japan's twentieth-century dietary transition by examining it from every major nutritional perspective. Although modern dietary transitions share a number of universal traits—declining intakes of staple carbohydrates, rising consumption of animal foods, and a greater variety of available foodstuffs are perhaps the three most notable shifts—they are less amenable to encompassing generalizations as far as the overall food energy supply is concerned.

In national statistics and international comparisons, this variable is usually expressed as an average daily per capita rate (normally in kcal per day rather than in standard energy units, that is, megajoules per day) that must be calculated by using the best available information about food production, trade, processing, and losses along the entire food chain. As difficult as this may be, the derivation of average daily per capita food supplies can be done fairly accurately wherever the relevant production and trade statistics are available. In contrast, reliable understanding of actual food consumption can come from only well-designed studies, and they are exceedingly rare.

When the primary statistics are available, it is possible to reconstruct (accurately or approximately, depending on the detail and quality of original data) food balance sheets for any particular period, and in the Japanese case these figures are readily available for the entire postwar period. That is why our review of the best available evidence for Japan's changing food supplies during the twentieth century, and particularly since the early 1950s, relies mostly on available food supply figures and why we augment the published statistics by our own calculations only for several key prewar years. While in most countries food supply derived from food balance sheets is the most reliable information available to follow the course of a dietary transition, Japan's unique set of regular food consumption surveys makes it possible to take a closer look at per capita food intakes for the entire postwar period. Consequently, when we look at individual foodstuffs in our examination of changing dietary patterns we can do so in terms of both average supply and typical per capita consumption.

The final section of this chapter looks at the interplay of Japan's traditional food preferences and modern nutritional choices—that is, the competition between and interaction of continuity and change in Japanese foodways. Japanese norms and food choices have changed profoundly, and in some cases even more rapidly than in the countries that have been historically more open to outside influences and new trends—and yet there is still so much that is unmistakably Japanese. The chapter closes with a brief appraisal of reverse flows, that is, major influences and impacts that the worldwide diffusion of Japanese cuisine and food preferences has had on Western diets. But before taking a systematic look at Japan's nutritional transformation, we summarize the factors behind the change.

Forces behind the Dietary Transition

As with any other complex process that unfolds across many decades, changes in a nation's diet are driven by many factors. Most of them are universal forces, but some are nation specific with few or no counterparts. And although the factors can be classified in such broad, distinct categories as economic development, advances in food production, universal dietary preferences, behavioral changes, or cultural preferences, even a cursory look at the history of dietary transitions will reveal their interdependence and many of their dynamic linkages (Caballero and Popkin 2002; Popkin 2003). Although it would be counterproductive to rank these factors, there is no doubt that the most important combination driving Japan's dietary transition has been that of rising disposable per capita income (resulting from decades of relatively strong economic growth) and the emergence of highly productive agricultural and animal husbandry practices (resulting from the universal adoption of high-

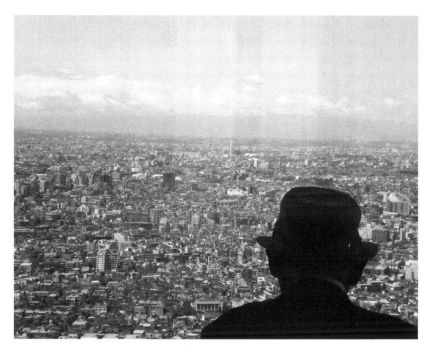

Figure 3.1
Two major forces behind Japan's dietary transition have been advancing urbanization and aging of the population. Here an old man looks at the capital's seemingly endless sprawl from the top of the city's municipal building. (V. Smil)

yielding crops and from mass production of meat, milk, and eggs by confined animals fed highly nutritious diets).

The first change gave consumers the means to follow different diets (with quality gains often as important as increases in the quantity of consumed foods), and the second set of advances made it possible to produce more than enough to satisfy the rising demand. In Japan's case, rising disposable incomes, increased farm production, and even higher productivity gains in U.S. agriculture, the leading source of Japan's food imports, combined to bring the average food cost of Japanese households from 66 percent of their total expenditures in 1946 to about 40 percent in the early 1960s and 23 percent by 2000, a share that was almost identical a decade later (Statistics Bureau 2011b). For comparison, EU shares are mostly between 12 and 15 percent, and Canadian and U.S. shares are below 10 percent (Eurostat 2011).

An important component of this economic growth is that, for most of the families, this advance has taken place as a result of rapid urbanization, a process that has not only improved disposable incomes but has led to important changes in household operation (above all, due to a much higher participation of women in the workforce), to easy access to ready-to-eat meals or to foods that require minimum home preparation. Exposure to new foods has been greatly accelerated by advancing economic globalization, the rising trade in foodstuffs (even the world's largest food producers have become major food importers), and mass-scale foreign travel that has helped to create demand for previously unobtainable foodstuffs.

Japan experienced continuous urbanization during the twentieth century, with the urban share of total population rising from less than 15 percent in 1900 to 40 percent by the early 1950s and nearly 80 percent by 2000. Female participation in the workforce, however, has not advanced as much as in many Western countries: by 2000, it was still only slightly above 40 percent. But travel abroad increased enormously after travel restrictions were lifted in 1964: the totals rose from just 168,000 in 1964 to about 2.5 million in 1975 and 17 million in 2000 (Mak, Carlile, and Dai 2004). These experiences have led to increased popularity of French, Italian, and Asian (Chinese, Indian, Thai, Indonesian) cuisine.

Every dietary transition is driven by universal (or nearly so) human preferences for certain kinds of nutrients and meals but it is not a simple across-the-board increase in the quantity or quality of traditional diets with no, or only a few, changes of their main components. While in the case of the poorest diets, increases in overall intakes of food energy were accompanied by similarly rising consumption of all macronutrients (carbohydrates, proteins, and fats), most cases of national dietary transition have seen rising food energy intake resulting from substantial shifts in the shares of key nutritional components. And these shifts have been primarily determined by widespread human preferences for eating more energy-dense diets in general, and more meat, lipids (of both plant and animal origin), and simple carbohydrates in particular (Smil 2002).

Declining demand for traditional grain staples has been the most common component of the modern dietary transition, driven by a combination of rising incomes, higher urbanization, and greater female workforce participation. The Japanese experience illustrates this shift perfectly: in affluent and urbanized Japan of the late 1990s, the cost of rice purchases fell below 5 percent of all household food expenses, it accounted for just over 1 percent of overall household outlays, and it contributed no more food energy than previously scarce meat. Kako (2004) showed that during the last two decades of the twentieth century, Japan's declining per capita rice consumption was correlated with higher overall expenditures, lower meat prices, population aging, and the share of income that women earned.

A number of comparisons show that this remarkable retreat from rice has been part of a universal income- and urbanization-driven trend. The Japanese trend has been mirrored by similar, or even faster, declines of rice demand in modernizing Thailand, Malaysia, South Korea, and China. During the four decades between 1965 and 2005, the share of food energy supplied by rice fell from 71 to 32 percent in Thailand, 47 to 22 percent in Malaysia, 48 to 30 percent in South Korea, and 37 to 26 percent in China compared to the drop from 43 to 23 percent in Japan. More recently, declining demand for rice can be also seen in Vietnam and Cambodia (International Rice Research Institute 2009b). Plotting these declining contributions against the rising economic performance shows that every tripling of per capita gross domestic product (expressed in purchasing parity terms) is accompanied by a 50 kg decrease in average annual per capita rice consumption (Smil 2005).

But the well-documented progress of Japan's dietary transition also illustrates another universal process: the eventual saturation of changing quantities and shares and, in some cases, their partial reversal, as well as the effect of specific dietary preferences. The rising energy density of urban diets, reflecting higher intakes of meat and animal and plant lipids is a universal hallmark of early stages of dietary transition that is followed by eventual saturation at levels that are influenced by specific dietary traditions. As a result, Japanese consumption of fatty meat, butter, and plant oils eventually leveled off and, in the case of lipids, at a much lower level than in other high-income countries, an exception explained by the relatively low level of overall food intakes and the traditional preference to eat meat in sliced or cut-up form. Cultural preference for seafood has also kept meat consumption from rising to levels common in even less affluent European countries. Clearly this particular saturation was not income limited because fish imports (above all, of tuna) have been even more costly.

Finally, it must be noted that the process of Japan's dietary transition received some important impulses, directly and indirectly, from the United States. Until 1952 it was Japan's occupying power and in that role closely supervised the country's affairs, and since then it has been the single most important ally and trading partner (both an admired and a denigrated one). The post-1945 expansion of whaling and the nation's uniquely high consumption of whale meat began directly with the decision of the Supreme Commander of the Allied Powers (SCAP) to promote the industry as an inexpensive means to secure more fat and protein for the energy-poor postwar diets. On November 30, 1945, SCAP authorized whaling in waters close to Japan—around the Bonin (Ogasawara Guntō) and Volcano Islands (Kazan Rettō)—and it reinstated Japanese Antarctic whaling in 1946 (Caprio and Sugita 2007).

The principal driver of rising milk consumption during the 1950s was the adoption of the national school lunch program, which started in elementary schools in 1952 and was clearly based on the U.S. National School Lunch Act of 1946 (Ralston et al. 2008). Besides a bread roll, margarine, and small side dishes of vegetables, fish, or whale meat, the lunch included a cup of milk, initially from powdered U.S. imports and later as fresh milk in bottles or cartons. Other obvious influences have ranged from the mass invasion of American fast food chains (both meaty and sweet: hamburgers as well as doughnuts) and convenience stores (especially the ubiquitous Lawson and Seven-Eleven) to the elevation of steaks and whiskies to high-status meals and alcoholic drinks.

The combination of universal and specific factors is behind the latest shifts in Japan's dietary intake. As in other affluent countries, a significant percentage of the aging population has become more health conscious, a concern that has been translated into falling consumption of lipids and fat-containing foodstuffs (whole milk, fatty meat) and lower sugar intake. But these trends go only so far: a large-scale study of the taste preferences of more than 29,000 Japanese adults found that significantly more people liked rather than disliked rich and heavy tastes, while the like and dislike shares were about even for sweet–tasting products (Matsushita et al. 2009).

Transformation of Food Supplies

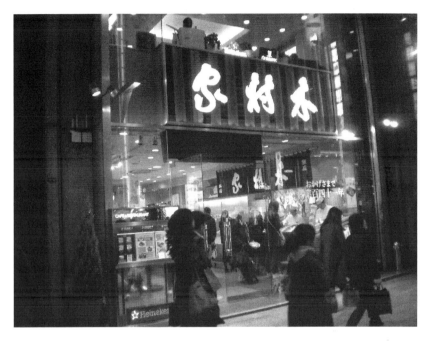

Figure 3.2
Modern Kimuraya bakery was rebuilt on the same spot in Tokyo's downtown where Kimura Yasubei opened the first Japanese-owned Western bakery in 1869. (V. Smil)

In the United States and Canada, as well as in the richest countries in Europe, food supply became more than adequate in gross energy terms during the nineteenth century, and the major effect of the twentieth-century dietary transition was on the composition of typical diets rather than on the overall quantity of digestible food energy. For example, U.S. historical data show average per capita food availability in 1909 (the earliest year for which the estimates are available) at 3,530 kcal per day compared to about 3,800 in 2000, an increase of only about 8 percent (Gortner 1975; Food and Agriculture Organization 2011a). In contrast, in nearly all modernizing countries, the qualitative changes in the composition of average diets have been accompanied by a notable increase of total food energy supply.

In Brazil the average per capita food supply rose from less than 2,200 kcal per day during the 1950s to 3,000 kcal per day by 2000 (a nearly 40 percent increase). In Indonesia the rise was even more impressive: from just above 1,700 kcal a day in 1960 to nearly 2,900 in 2000, a 70 percent rise in just two generations. Because of its history, China offers an even more extreme example. During the world's worst, and overwhelmingly man-made (specifically Mao-made), famine, more than 30 million people died as average per capita food energy supply dropped to below 1,600 kcal a day (Smil 1999). Even after the country emerged from this catastrophe, inefficient collectivized Maoist agriculture could produce only enough food to keep the country barely above the subsistence level: average food energy supply was barely above 2,000 kcal a day in 1970.

De facto privatization of farming, the key component of Deng Xiaoping's economic reforms, changed this situation rapidly. China became a net food exporter in 1985 as its average per capita food availability reached 2,600 kcal a day; by 1990 the country's per capita food energy supply was just 5 percent below the Japanese level; and by 2000 China averaged more for every one of its 1.26 billion citizens than did Japan: nearly 3,000 versus about 2,800 kcal a day. In contrast to these two patterns of change, some notable shifts in the composition of the average diet in Japan's dietary transition have not been accompanied by any substantial increases of overall food energy supply. In terms of macronutrient supply, Japan's dietary transition has conformed to the three key universal expectations (average diets have experienced falling shares of complex carbohydrates and rising shares of sugar and animal protein), but it has also retained two important unique characteristics thanks to much less pronounced increases in the intake of lipids and sugar.

The best way to trace the long-term trends of Japan's food supplies is by selecting specific years for closer examination. The best available data on crop, livestock, and seafood production and on agricultural trade for those years serve as our inputs into the reconstruction of pre–World War II food balance sheets while the postwar food balances are available from Japan's Ministry of Agriculture, Forestry and Fisheries (2011) as well as from the U.N.'s Food and Agriculture Organization (2011a). In 1900 we get a glimpse of a still overwhelmingly traditional agroecosystem during the closing years of the Meiji era, in many ways an easily recognizable descendant of the two and a half centuries of Tokugawa rule. The mid-1920s were a time of slowly improving food availability and nutritional quality, and a decade later, the country had become a major importer of rice from its colonies. In 1950 Japan not yet recovered from the destruction of World War II, and the lingering food shortages of the postwar years were not sufficiently overcome until the mid-1950s.

By the mid-1950s, when Japan had finally surpassed its prewar economic performance, its rather traditional food supply was about to undergo major changes. By 1965, Japan was rapidly shifting some of its traditional foodways, and a decade later its food supply had largely moved into a new consumption pattern of what might be called incipient affluence. By 1990, when Japan stood at the apex of its economic achievement (Smil 2009), its newly found affluence and the belated opening to substantial agricultural imports had basically accomplished Japan's dietary transition. The decades-long process had largely run its course, and the situation at the start of the millennium, and still today, is not dissimilar to that in 1990.

Food Balance Sheets

Determining how much food a nation has available for human consumption requires constructing food balance sheets for a calendar year. In countries with detailed and reliable statistics, that is a relatively straightforward task, albeit one that cannot be done without some simplifying assumptions. National food balance sheets encompass domestic production, as well as the net trade of all important plant and animal foodstuffs. If such numbers are relatively large, they might include changes in stocks. All advanced economies publish such accounts on a regular basis and forward them to the Food and Agriculture Organization to be used in its worldwide compendium.

Preparation of food balance sheets requires many specific adjustments that should use the latest information. For crops this includes subtracting amounts used for seed, industrial conversions (most often for alcoholic beverages and starch), livestock feeding, and (usually the least reliable component) waste during storage, processing, and transportation. The net result of these adjustments is the amount of domestically produced and imported plant biomass that is available to be consumed directly or to undergo processing. In the latter case, appropriate extraction rates for milling of cereals, pressing of oil seeds, or production of sugar or bean curd must be used in order to derive actual supply of individual plant foodstuffs.

Preparation of the animal food component of food balance sheets begins with information on the number and typical live weights of slaughtered animals and on net meat imports, with meat production expressed (most often) in terms of carcass weight (excluding slaughtering fats and putting edible offal into a separate category) or (less often) in terms of only edible fraction (meat, animal fat, offal). Milk and egg outputs and aquatic catches and aquacultural products are taken from available statistics and must be corrected for the net trade and adjusted for processing losses, nonfood uses (mostly as fish meals and fish oils used for animal feeding), and waste. Annual mass totals for individual foodstuffs can then be expressed as average per capita supply rates (kg/ year) and converted to the total food energy supply (usually kcal or megajoules per day) as well as to the contributions of principal macronutrients (carbohydrates, proteins, and lipids in grams per day).

Unfortunately, these average per capita rates of food supply derived from food balance sheets are commonly mistaken for actual food consumption. If that were true, then Americans and the citizens of many EU countries would have to eat, on average, 3,500 to 3,800 kcal of food every day, impossibly high intakes that would imply (given the fact that actual intakes for infants, young children, and very old people are much below 2,000 kcal a day) adult food consumption in excess of 4,500 or 5,000 kcal a day. Food balance sheets do not tell us how much people eat—only how much food is available during a given year. In modern economies (where only negligible shares of food are produced by households for their own consumption), food balance sheets inform us about food supply at wholesale levels. They should be never mistaken for actual food intakes, but when they are prepared by using consistent procedures, they can be used for revealing historical and international comparisons.

Several studies have attempted to reconstruct Japan's food balance sheets for selected years during the closing decades of the nineteenth and the first half of the twentieth centuries, with some reconstructions going as far back as 1874, the first year for which some crop and livestock production statistics are available (Nasu 1927; Nakamura 1966;

Nakayama 1967; Kaneda 1970; Hayami and Yamada 1970; Mosk and Pak 1978). There are four major problems with these reconstructions: early crop production statistics are considerably more unreliable than the latter data; different number of commodities were included in the preparation of food balance sheets; supply of wild nonstaple foods (vegetables, mushrooms, wild animals) can be only estimated; and the typical multipliers used to convert harvested crops into foodstuffs are often uncertain.

Available Food Energy

For the year 1900, the lowest rate published in the sources listed in the preceding paragraph is 1,948 kcal/capita and the highest one is 2,445 kcal, a difference of 20 percent, while the mean of all calculated values is 2,132 kcal. The range is narrower for 1925, with extremes at 2,046 and 2,374 kcal/capita, a gap of 13 percent, and a mean of 2,216 kcal. We have used unadjusted official crop and livestock production statistics corrected for appropriate amounts of net foreign trade in agricultural products and nonfood uses (mainly for seed) in order to prepare yet another approximate food balance sheet reconstruction for those two years and ended up (using conservative assumptions) with about 2,100 kcal in 1900 and 2,200 kcal in 1925 (table 3.1; graph 3.1). Average per capita food supply calculated for 1935 was also about 2,200 kcal a day. Starting in 1948, food balance sheet calculations are available from the official Japanese statistics.

The first seven years of these figures are problematic because they show average daily food supply 140 to 280 kcal below the actual intake, an impossibility explained (at least for the earliest year) by the existence of a substantial black market. Assuming that very little food was wasted during those years of serious food shortages, the best solution is to use the intake totals instead. The rate for 1950 was thus about 2,100 kcal a day, no better than in 1900 and lower than during the 1930s. By 1965 the mean supply had risen to 2,450 kcal a day, and in 1990 it was just over 2,600 kcal, almost exactly the same rate that prevailed in 2000. However, all of these rates are 5 to 8 percent lower than those in the FAO's (2011a) food balance sheets. These differences arise from different assumptions regarding food processing, losses, and nonfood uses.

Any discrepancies of less than 5 percent might be dismissed as unavoidable. On the other hand, the smallest difference (about 120 kcal) is nearly

Table 3.1
Average per capita food supply and intake, 1900–2008

Year	Average daily supply (kcal/capita)	Shares (percent) contributed by			Average daily per capita intake			
		Carbohydrates	Proteins	Lipids	Energy (kcal)	Protein (grams)	Lipids (grams)	Carbohydrates (grams)
1900	2,100	80	11	9	2,050	63	15	420
1925	2,200	80	11	9	2,100	68	18	420
1935	2,200	79	12	9	2,100	68	18	420
1950	2,100	79	13	8	2,100	68	18	420
1975	2,540	63	15	22	2,226	81	55	340
1990	2,610	60	15	25	2,026	79	57	290
2000	2,610	57	15	27	1,948	78	57	270
2008	2,473	57	16	27	1,867	78	56	260

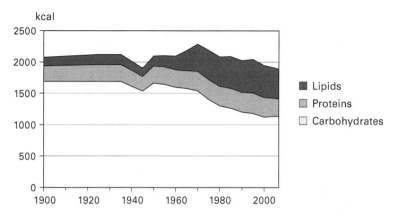

Graph 3.1
Daily food energy intake and its constituents, 1900–2008.

twice as large as the recent average daily per capita supply of all fruits, while the largest difference (about 210 kcal) is about 15 percent higher than the average daily per capita supply of all meat. For the postwar years, we use the average food availability figures prepared by the Ministry of Agriculture, Forestry and Fisheries and slightly rounded to the nearest 10 kcal and the nearest gram of protein and fat (table 3.1). Japan has been through five distinct periods in terms of its overall food energy supply. The first, and the longest one, was one of low and only marginally improving availability of food energy during the first four decades of the twentieth century, with average per capita supplies ranging between just 2,100 and 2,200 kcal per day. This was followed by roughly a decade of barely adequate food supply, first due to falling food availability during the last three years of the war, then to serious postwar food shortages in 1946 and 1947, followed by another five years of limited food supply.

Only in 1948 did the average per capita supply go above 2,100 kcal, and only in 1956 it did surpass 2,200 kcal a day, the rate that had been reached by the mid-1920s. Afterward came two decades of rising food energy availability to nearly 2,600 kcal a day by the mid-1970s. The fourth period, between the mid-1970s and the mid-1990s, saw a small rise to a bit above 2,600 kcal. Since that time, Japan's food supply has declined slightly, slipping below 2,600 kcal a day by 2004 and averaging just above 2,500 kcal a day by 2007 (Statistics Bureau 2011a). This means that Japan's overall food energy supply remains considerably lower than in other affluent nations. The FAO put Japan's per capita supply for 2005 (the last year for which FAO's worldwide food balance sheets are available; we present the totals rounded to the nearest 10 kcal) was 2,740 kcal a day compared to 3,160 kcal in Russia, close to 3,500 calories for the EU, and 3,860 kcal in the United States. More notably, in that year, Japan's average availability of food energy was not only below that of Brazil (3,120 kcal) but also of China (2,970 kcal), although those two countries had lower shares of protein derived from animal foodstuffs—about 15 percent less in Brazil and a third less in China.

Trends in Food Intakes

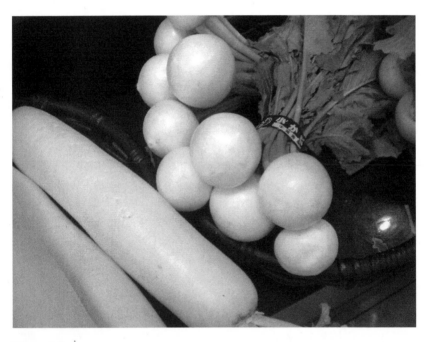

Figure 3.3
Food trends come and go, but many constants remain: white radishes (*daikon*) are the mainstay of Japan's pickled food accompaniments (*tsukemono*). (V. Smil)

In order to find the actual average per capita food consumption, the totals in the food balance sheet approach must be reduced by losses that take place before the food available at the wholesale level reaches households (due to storage, transportation and retailing), by household waste (due to spoilage, food preparation and cooking), and by unconsumed leftovers. Given the wide variety of foodstuffs and widely differing methods and standards of their storage, handling, and transportation procedures, it is not surprising that there are no comprehensive figures regarding typical annual postharvest food losses. This means that it is impossible to prepare a reasonably representative equivalent of a food balance sheet that would provide fairly reliable information on how much has actually been eaten. Economists have often used information on food quantities derived from income and expenditure surveys, but this approach entirely misses all postretail food losses. The best understanding of actual consumption thus comes only from food surveys.

If they are to be representative, such surveys must examine thousands of consumers, and if they are to be as accurate as possible, they should be administered or supervised by trained personnel. Both of these requirements are costly, and that is why most national food intake surveys rely on a subject's recall of foods eaten during the previous day, an expedient but questionable approach. As already noted, Japan is a notable exception: its National Health and Nutrition Survey is conducted by registered dietitians, and other health professionals conduct the associated physical examination. The intake survey relies primarily on the combination of weighing actual amounts of foods before or after preparation (or both times) as well as the amounts left or wasted and recording the meals where weighing is impossible (e.g., when eating out). Staff dietitians provide guidance on how to monitor these intakes, note the frequency of meals and eating and living habits (including physical activity, sleep, drinking, and smoking), check records, and resolve any problems.

The survey began amid severe food shortages in Tokyo in 1945, instigated by the General Headquarters of the U.S. occupation forces in order to ascertain the need for emergency food imports. Its coverage expanded during the next two years, and by 1948 it was nationwide. Between 1946 and 1963, the survey was conducted four times a year on three consecutive days, and since 1995 it has been just a single-day affair of collecting data from more than 12,000 people in about 5,000 randomly selected households (Katanoda and Matsumura 2002). Differences in the timing of the survey, its frequency, and its coverage do not make its result perfectly comparable, but a close look makes it clear that none of these shortcomings has any fundamentally detrimental effect on the outcome and that the survey's results can be used as a remarkably reliable record to assess more than six decades of changing average per capita food consumption. Katanoda et al. (2005) had also found that the study well represents the entire population, having only 1 to 2 percent more females and a very slight rural bias.

Food Energy

With these reassurances, we can make some fairly conclusive judgments about the postwar trends in Japan's food consumption and the specific nature of the country's long-term dietary transition. We start with aggregate values before moving to individual components.

While the average per capita supply of food energy rose by about 25 percent during the twentieth century (from about 2,100 kcal in 1900 to around 2,600 kcal a day in 2000), actual food intake showed a modest (less than 15 percent) increase until the early 1970s (from about 2,000 kcal in 1900 to nearly 2,300 kcal between 1971 and 1973) followed by a gradual decline to less than 2,000 kcal (1,948) by the year 2000 (table 3.1; graph 3.1). This downward trend continued during the first decade of the twenty-first century, bringing the mean per capita intake to just below 1,900 kcal by 2007 (Statistics Bureau 2011a).

Japan's average per capita food energy consumption is thus now less than in 1900, but there is nothing puzzling or surprising about this fact once it is put into context: human energy requirements are a complex function of basal metabolism, growth, and prevailing physical activity, and food supply is a key factor in determining body growth. Basal metabolism (the energy needed per unit of body mass) shows an exponential decline with age after reaching maturity and significant individual departures from an expected population mean, while the share of energy needed for body growth is obviously highest in early childhood and becomes minimal (for tissue repairs) after puberty (Smil 2008). Physical activity in the adult population depends on the stage of economic development, and it also declines with age, and people living with a chronically suboptimal food supply will not be able to express their full growth potential.

In 1900 Japan was a demographically young society with children and young adults greatly outnumbering people over sixty years of age. Its average basal energy and body growth needs were obviously higher (mainly due to larger shares of teenagers and people in their twenties) than in today's aging population. Moreover, in 1900 Japan was a predominantly agricultural economy reliant on physical labor, with draft animals contributing much less to fieldwork than they did in Europe and even in some parts of China at the beginning of the twentieth century. Hence the typical adult food needs were higher than in a modern society where most jobs are either sedentary or require only moderate exertion. Because there is no likely way to reverse either the aging or the mechanization trend, we must expect Japan's future average per capita food energy consumption to remain below 2,000 kcal a day.

At the same time, food supply during the late Meiji era was insufficient to meet not only all basal energy and physical activity needs but also growth requirements, and that is why most Japanese remained stunted. Japan's historical statistics (table 24-3 of the online edition at http://www.stat.go.jp/english/data/chouki/24.htm) contain a series of anthropometric data on average body height and mass measured annually at mostly two-year age intervals between ages six and twenty-four. Although this series has some sample bias and some lapses in coverage, it shows a remarkable transition from stunting to full growth potential. The average height of twenty-year old males increased from 160.9 centimeters in 1900 to 164.5 centimeters by 1939, and after temporary wartime stunting, the resumed growth brought the average height to 171.8 centimeters by 2000. The average weight gain for the same age group was about 23 percent, from 53 to 65.4 kg. Of course, better nutrition was not the only factor behind these gains: better housing, less strenuous work, and disease prevention have also contributed.

Protein
This growth could not have been realized without higher consumption of better-quality proteins, an improvement that is not captured by comparing overall food energy intakes: they could have come mostly from staple carbohydrates whose low-quality proteins would not have had the same effect as did the intakes of animal proteins with their ideal proportions of the essential amino acids required for human growth. All proteins, plant and animal, have the nine essential amino acids required by human metabolism in order to produce our body proteins, but no plant proteins have the ideal ratio of these amino acids. Most important, all

cereal proteins (in wheat, rice, and corn) are deficient in lysine, and leguminous proteins (in peas, beans, lentils, and soybeans) have suboptimal amounts of methionine. Careful combination of cereal and leguminous foods can satisfy the overall protein requirements, but it is easier, and for most people also more enjoyable, to consume animal foodstuffs with their perfect proteins.

In 1900 Japan's overall protein intake was suboptimal in both absolute and qualitative terms. Although at least one historical reconstruction puts its daily intake as high as 67 to 69 grams per day (Nakamura 1966), a more realistic rate would be no more than 60, and perhaps as little as 55, grams per day (11 percent of all energy). By 1925 the daily rate had risen well above 60 grams per day, but it did not, as Mosk and Pak (1978) estimated, reach nearly 75 grams per day: that level was reached only in the modernizing Japan of the mid-1960s. The first official postwar data for 1946 show average protein intake at only about 59 grams per day (about 13 percent of all food energy), rates between 69 and 70 grams per day prevailed between 1952 and 1963, the peak was reached with about 84 grams per day in 1973, and this was followed by fluctuating intakes, mostly between 79 and 81 grams per day, until 1998 (or about 15 percent of all food energy). Afterward came a substantial decline to only to 70 grams per day by 2005 (table 3.1).

In 1900 less than 3 percent of all food energy was of animal origin. By 1950 that share was still no higher than 5 percent, but then it surpassed 10 percent by 1963 and 20 percent by 1977, and it has been at about 25 percent since the mid-1990s. This means that animal proteins accounted for less than 15 percent of the total in 1900. Because of relatively high intakes of staple grains, overall protein consumption was not inadequate even during the late 1940s, when less than 20 percent of protein came from animal foods. That share rose to 25 percent by 1950, surpassed 50 percent by 1981, and reached about 55 percent in 2000. Both the average (around 80 grams per day) and animal protein (around 45 grams per day) intake thus remain below the world's highest levels (those in the United States and France, which are around 100 grams per day, with at least 60 percent coming from animal foods), but they have been well above the requirements for vigorous childhood and adolescent growth and for active and healthy life, and there would be no advantage in raising them.

Fats and Carbohydrates

There were two main reasons for the traditionally low consumption of lipids in general and animal fats in particular: limited cultivation of oil seeds (rapeseed and sesame), which, unlike European olives, had to be grown on land suitable for cereals, and the already noted very low consumption of animal foods. Consumption of lipids remained negligible (less than 20 grams per day, supplying no more than 10 percent of food energy) until the early 1950s, but then it nearly tripled in thirty years to almost 60 grams per day by the early 1980s, with animal fats supplying roughly half of the total. The average fat intakes stayed at that level until the late 1990s, but with a more health-conscious aging population, they have subsequently declined to less than 55 grams per day. The latest surveys indicate that adults over twenty years of age derive about 25 percent of their food energy from fats and that, surprisingly, females eat proportionately more lipids than men do. In 2006, 48 percent of females had diets with a fat-to-energy ratio below 25 percent, and about 27 percent consumed food with more than 30 percent of food energy from fat. The comparable statistics for males, respectively, were nearly 60 percent and only about 18 percent (Ministry of Health, Labour and Welfare 2009).

Although Japanese like fatty foodstuffs, they consume them in smaller quantities and less frequently than most Europeans and Americans do, so in the average Japanese diet, no more than 25 to 27 percent of all food energy comes from lipids (graph 3.1), the lowest share among all affluent countries. Nearly all rich nations of North America and Europe have nationwide fat energy ratio above 30 percent (Centers for Disease Control 2004; Ocké et al. 2009). Rising shares of food energy derived from protein and lipid consumption had to lower the share of energy supplied by carbohydrates. In absolute terms average Japanese carbohydrate intakes fell from more than 400 grams per day during the early 1950s to only about 270 grams per day by 2000, and in relative terms, their share of food energy declined from close to 80 percent during the first half of the twentieth century to about 57 percent by 2000. But the sources of these carbohydrates have changed little in relative terms: in the early 1950s, cereals supplied about 85 percent, and by 2000 their share was still about 82 percent.

Until the early 1960s, the Japanese food supply was thus even lower, and it was even more dominated by carbohydrates and contained even less fat and less animal protein than in Spain, Italy, or Greece, the paragons of frugal, high-carbohydrate, low-fat Mediterranean diets. Because of the lack of regular food intake surveys, the comparison can be based on only food supply (not on actual intakes) derived from the food balance sheet. The result shows that in 1961, Japan's food energy supply averaged less than 2,500 kcal a day, with 60 percent of it from cereals and less than 4 percent from plant and animal lipids; the shares, respectively, for Italy were about 2,900, 44 percent, and 13 percent; for Spain, just over 2,600, 40 percent, and 13 percent; and for Greece, a bit more than 2,800, 47 percent, and 16 percent.

Micronutrients

Japan's annual nutritional surveys also monitor the intake of several micronutrients. Between 1946 and 2000, average daily intakes of calcium and vitamin A and vitamin B_2 more than doubled. The first rise was largely the result of a relatively high consumption of dairy products (graph 3.2), a major departure from the traditional diet. The second increase came mostly from higher consumption of eggs and red and orange fruits and vegetables (published vitamin A intakes for the years 1946 to 1954 were exaggerated due to incorrect food composition data, so the comparisons should start only with 1955). During the same period, intake of vitamin B_1 (thiamine) declined by 35 percent, most likely due to falling consumption of grains. Per capita intake of vitamin C was put at nearly 190 milligrams per day in 1946, and this was followed by a rapid decline and rebound, with the latest rates at about 100 milligrams per day. These are puzzling trends given the generally rising consumption of vegetables, fruits, and fruit juices; the best explanation attributes it to to falling consumption of leafy green vegetables, but in any case, average intakes of 100 milligrams per day are quite adequate.

Data for salt intake, a matter of concern in the traditionally highly salty Japanese diet, have been available only since 1973, and they showed no great shifts until 2000, remaining mostly between 12 and 13 milligrams per day, still above the maximum amount of 10 milligrams per day recommended by Japanese health authorities, with intakes higher in northern Japan and lower in Kansai (western Japan). Falling consumption of traditionally very salty *tsukemono* is a major contributor to this

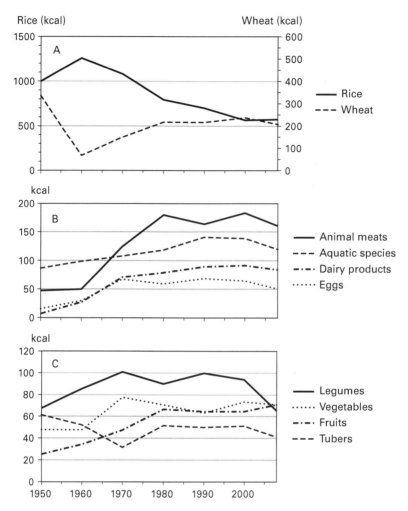

Graph 3.2
Changes in daily energy intake of major foodstuffs: cereals (A), animal products (B),
and other vegetable products (C), 1950–2008.

latest trend: many varieties have become less salty, reflecting consumers'
concern over high salt intakes. Remarkably for an island country, the
bulk of Japan's salt consumption is imported: in 2000 less than 15
percent of the total supply came from Japanese producers (mostly from
ion-exchange systems) and the rest from imports of mostly sun-dried salt
(Salt Industry Center of Japan 2009).

Japanese Foodways: Continuity and Change

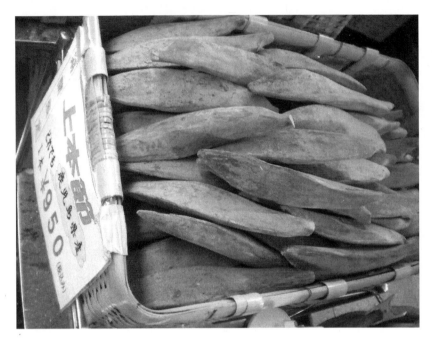

Figure 3.4
Elaborately prepared *katsuobushi* is an excellent illustration of the durability of many of Japan's traditional foodways. (V. Smil)

Assessing the relative importance of continuity and change is a constant challenge in providing sensible historical perspectives, whether dealing with the modernization of political regimes or dietary patterns. Balanced accounts are often elusive: selective inattention to realities that might complicate an appealing (hence often simplistic) interpretation, biased approaches to unruly realities, personal experiences and attitudes (science is never immune to those), and prevailing opinions (which inevitably change with time) can produce conclusions that might not be entirely wrong but are far from often contradictory and nuanced realities.

Offering a balanced appraisal of contemporary Japanese food consumption, the outcome of both extensive and intensive dietary transition, is a perfect embodiment of these challenges. Continuity and tradition seem to be everywhere, deep seated, evident in everyday choices and acts— but so are the imported foodstuffs and the ways of eating that were entirely foreign just a few generations ago and are now seen as completely Japanese. In so many ways, modern Japanese foodways are clearly beholden to the customs and traditions of the Tokugawa period, particularly its last three pre-1860s generations: the diet of the Edo period remains the foundation of Japanese culinary culture (Harada 2008; Watanabe 2004). At the same time, Western dietary influences have been pervasive and are particularly entrenched among the young adults of the post-1980 generation and among adolescents and children. Foreigners encountering Japan for the first time (and some of them every time they return or for as long as they stay) are enchanted by this coexistence, indeed a fusion, of the two worlds.

They admire the spectrum of foodstuffs ranging from an unmatched abundance of traditionally favorite seafood species (from squid to tuna) and artfully presented *nigirizushi* and *wagashi* to no less appealing French pastries and choice fruit from around the world. But a different interpretation is possible. Shizuo Tsuji, a leading chef of the first postwar generation, offered a distinctly unflattering appraisal of Japan's modern cuisine, sparing neither its traditional foundation nor its imported component (Tsuji 1980, 23):

The foreign dishes have been denatured to suit the Japanese palate, and, I am sorry to say, our own cuisine is no longer authentic. It has been polluted with frozen foods, which are freely used in heedless ignorance of tradition. Japan must be the only country in the world where the everyday fare is such a hodgepodge, and whose people know so little about their own traditional cuisine that they do not try to preserve its authenticity.

Perhaps Tsuji can be judged too much a purist, but there is no doubt that the fusion (or hodgepodge) has progressed tremendously since he wrote that opinion three decades ago. After all, Japan is now a country where no other food store has more locations (more than 12,000) or higher annual sales (approaching $20 billion) than Seven-Eleven, with its mixture of Western and Japanese foodstuffs. And the country's leading fast food restaurant is not dispensing *soba* or *onigiri*. McDonald's has nearly 4,000 stores around the country, its annual sales now surpass $5 billion, and it fosters a dietary hodgepodge by offering such items as shrimp and teriyaki burgers and green tea-flavored milkshakes.

Japan is also a country where a mixture of rice and a thick curry sauce (at home usually made from solid or powdered package of roux), known as *karē raisu*, is a national favorite. A 2008 survey of 400 unmarried adults in their twenties found that *karē raisu* was the favorite choice for an evening meal, well ahead of pasta and spaghetti, stir-fried vegetables, fried rice, and salad (Norinchukin Bank 2008). And when in 2008 baseball star Ichirō Suzuki revealed that he eats *karē raisu* for breakfast on his game days, supermarkets began to sell *asa karē* (morning curry) packages.

Value judgments about the relative merits of tradition and modernity will be always strongly influenced by personal preferences and experiences, but Japan's excellent postwar statistics make it possible to appraise the two contending trends of dietary tradition and nutritional innovation in a dispassionate manner. A minor problem is selecting a starting point for such historical comparisons. Nationwide food intake studies have been available since 1947, but during that year, Japan's food supply was still anomalously low and clearly unrepresentative of the normal diet. By 1950 the situation was still far from normal, but by 1955, the country's standard of living and supply of food had surpassed the best prewar achievements.

We will compare the weight of individual diet components (in grams) consumed per capita per day as well as the total food energy (in kcal per day in the original statistics) supplied by different food categories. Finally, there must be arbitrary cutoffs for classifying a shift as a minor fluctuation (including the inevitable errors in gathering and converting the intake data and their long-term intercomparability), a significant change, or a transformational development. We use 10 percent for the first instance, 10 to 25 percent for the second one, and more than 25 percent to identify the last category.

Rapid Change and Continuity of Intakes

Using these criteria, there is only one principal component of Japan's average diet that has undergone less than a transformational change between 1950 and 2000: vegetable intakes were up by only some 15 percent at the same time that the daily weight of all other principal foodstuffs consumed per capita was down or up by more than 25 percent. The declines were 46 percent for cereals (50 percent for rice) and 49 percent for tubers, and the increases ranged from 25 percent for wheat and 50 percent for seafood all the way to some very large multiples: almost three times as much fruit, roughly seven times more eggs, almost nine and a half times as much meat, and nearly nineteen times as much milk and dairy products (graph 3.2).

And if the increases were calculated using the respective maxima reached during the 1980s or 1990s (before the intakes began to fall), relative shifts for some foodstuffs would be even higher: a 3.2-fold increase for foods of animal origin (the peak in 1995) and a 10-fold increase of meat consumption (the peak in 1981). In terms of principal nutrients, there was hardly any change in the overall intake of protein, while the consumption of lipids had nearly tripled. For comparison, the best available long-term statistics for the U.S. per capita supply of major foodstuffs show that between 1909 (the earliest year for which the data are available) and 2006, cereals and dairy products were down by, respectively, 35 percent and 43 percent, while fish was up by 26 percent and meat by 25 percent. In terms of macronutrients, there were 12 percent and 14 percent declines for total protein and carbohydrates, respectively, and a 40 percent rise for lipids (U.S. Bureau of the Census 1975; U.S. Department of Agriculture 2008). The only large multiple was for chicken, a slightly more than sixfold rise in a century.

This means that the average Japanese diet had seen more profound relative changes during the fifty years after 1950 or 1955 than the American diet did during nearly the century between 1909 and 2006. Evidence is clear: as far as the relative shifts in the daily intakes of major foodstuffs are concerned, the Japanese diet of the second half of the twentieth century was characterized more by change than by continuity. This leaves us with the only (but critically important) variable as the marker of Japan's dietary continuity: average per capita intake of all food energy. This rate stood (rounding to the nearest 10) at 2,100 kcal in 1950 as well as in 1955, it peaked at 2,280 kcal in 1972, and then it declined to 1,950 kcal in 2000 and 1,900 kcal in 2005.

The last two rates were obviously influenced by the progressive aging of Japan's population, the process characterized by falling basal metabolic rates as well as declining energy requirements for physical activity. The peaks of food energy intake during the early 1970s were due to the combination of a relatively vigorous population growth of the preceding generation (the average was well over 1 percent between 1950 and 1975, compared to 0.2 percent in 2000, creating additional food energy needs for pregnancy, lactation, and child and adolescent growth) and for physical labor in expanding manufacturing and construction industries. This means that the changing intakes have closely followed the shifts in population structure and activity needs, and they have also remained close to the expected food energy requirements calculated on the basis of the most appropriate basal metabolic, growth, and activity needs.

Given the paucity of reliable food intake data, it is not easy to make revealing international comparisons. The most extensive survey of adult European food intakes (part of a large-scale prospective study about cancer and nutrition that was based on standardized twenty-four-hour dietary recall) showed that between 1995 and 2000, the average adult male (between thirty-five and seventy-four years of age) intakes ranged from lows of around 2,400 kcal per day in Sweden to 2,700 kcal per day in Spain, with German averages around 2,500 kcal per day and Italian and Danish means above 2,600 kcal per day (Ocké et al. 2009). Averages from the U.S. National Health and Nutrition Examination Survey (NHANES; also based on dietary recall) for the years 1995 to 2000 were about 2,800 kcal a day for males between twenty and thirty-nine years of age, and 2,600 kcal a day for men between forty and fifty-nine years (Wright et al. 2003). In contrast, Japan's 1995 mean for men between thirty and sixty-nine years of age was about 2,300 kcal a day and in 2000 a bit less, about 2,250 kcal per day, and the intakes were thus significantly (10–15 percent) below those of European and American adults.

Comparable rates for females ranged from about 1,650 calories a day in Greece to about 1,950 kcal day in France, with German, Italian, and Swedish rates between 1,800 and 1,900 kcal a day, and the U.S. averages for women aged twenty to thirty-nine years just over 2,000 kcal day. For women forty to fifty-nine years of age, they were just above 1,800 kcal a day. Japanese female averages were mostly between 1,850 and 1,900 kcal a day for ages thirty to sixty-nine in 1995 and just above 1,800 kcal a day in 2000. This means that at the century's end, the average food energy intakes of Japanese females were very similar to the U.S. rates and that they also broadly overlapped with European means. But how do these conclusions square with the high obesity rates in the United States and Europe? If U.S .males consume daily only 10 to 15 percent more food energy than do their Japanese counterparts and if the female intakes in the two countries are similar, why is the Japanese obesity rate an order of magnitude lower? And why the European countries, with food intakes much closer to the U.S. means, also have significantly lower obesity rates than does North America?

Four major factors explain this puzzle. The first one is a common underreporting of food intake in dietary recall surveys, the only source of information on population-wide food consumption in the United States and Europe. It is almost certain that the actual intakes are significantly higher. Second, even a small excess of food energy intakes translates over time into substantial weight gains if the difference between energy inflow and outflow is chronic, as it clearly is in North America and in large parts of Europe. Third, low levels of physical activity have become the norm for most Western populations, which aggravates this accumulation process.

And, finally, food energy inputs may be easily reducible to a common denominator, but dietary calories are not equal. Different compositions of typical food intakes, with much higher shares of fats and simple sugars in Western diets in general and in America's consumption in particular, account for the seemingly minor difference in overall intakes of energy. Moreover, an analysis of fifty-five years of Japanese anthropometric data demonstrated that (in a dramatic contrast to recent rapid increases of obesity among comparable Western cohorts) isochrones for the body mass index of those five to seventeen years old remained almost horizontal between 1948 and 2003 (Hermanussen et al. 2007). This lack of evidence for obesity increase during more than half a century that coincided with major dietary changes suggests that Japanese children and adolescents may not be as easily affected by a number of environmental factors that have been identified as the major drivers of the rising prevalence of Western obesity.

At the same time, longer-term prospects may look decidedly different as some local and nationwide surveys show an increasing prevalence of obesity among elementary school boys and girls (Yoshinaga et al. 2003), proportionately higher intakes of fats and animal protein than in adults, and lack of daily physical exercise (Murata 2000). And a study of junior high school students identified major associations with adolescent overweight that are well known from Western settings: parental overweight, skipping breakfast, eating quickly, long hours of TV watching and video game playing, physical inactivity, and not enough sleep (Sun et al. 2009).

Other Continuities

Tracing the post-1950 rise and fall of major food groups shows more change than continuity, but this grand pattern of change hides many constants. Many individual foodstuffs that were traditionally highly regarded have retained their favorite status, and many common food-ways have remained highly popular and fairly resistant to change. The first one of the four most notable components belonging to the first category is a continuing preference for a variety of foodstuffs and dishes to be consumed concurrently rather than in any specific set order; the second one could be best labeled as undiminished aquatic omnivory; the third one is the lasting preferences for raw, or minimally cooked, food; and the fourth one is the attention given to food presentation.

The first habit was noted during the first encounters between the Japanese and the Americans. After Commodore Perry gave formal banquets on board of his ship, he wrote in his accounts how "in the eagerness of the Japanese appetite, there was but little discrimination in the choice of dishes and in the order of courses, and the most startling heterodoxy was exhibited in the confusing commingling of fish, flesh, and fowl, soups and syrups, fruits and fricassees, roast and boiled, pickles and preserves" (Perry 1856, 375).

This fondness for fusion and a frequent absence of specific eating order is encapsulated every day in a multitude of compartmentalized Japanese *bentō*, with their variety of often artfully presented ingredients and with no set order for their consumption (Kamekura, Watanabe, and Bosker 1989; Ekuan 1998). There are no generally accepted or highly preferred guidelines for *bentō* composition. An old 4:3:2:1 rule (four parts of rice; three parts of fish, meat, or meat substitute; two parts of vegetables; and one part of pickles) is as valid as splitting the content between rice and a few *okazu* dishes and, in any case, such rules do not dictate the order of eating.

By far the most impressive display of Japan's aquatic omnivory is a visit to Tsukiji, the world's largest market for aquatic products (Bestor 2004). Tokyo's main fish market was moved to this location along the Sumida River from downtown (at Nihonbashi) after the 1923 earth-quake, and since the 1970s, its activities have greatly expanded with Japan's rising seafood imports. Every day the market handles scores of species ranging from frozen tuna flown in from around the world to boxes of sea urchins and brilliantly colored fish eggs. Other displays of this traditional omnivory can be seen in the continuing popularity of seasonally available seafood, of both the simplest and inexpensive kind (broiled eels, *kabayaki*, in summer) and elaborately prepared and expensive springtime eating of translucent slices of *fugu*, as well as in nostalgic craving of some older people for a slice of whale meat.

Japanese preference for eating raw foods extends beyond the two iconic choices of seafood, *sashimi* and sushi. Chicken (*torisashi*), beef (*gyūsashi*), and horse meat (*basashi*) can be eaten as *sashimi*, and for a traditional breakfast, a raw eggs is cracked on top of boiled rice (*tamago-kake gohan*). Nevertheless, some kinds of sushi are never eaten raw: conger eel (*anago*) is first simmered in sweet sauce, shrimp (*ebi*) is boiled, and mackerel (*saba*) is marinated in vinegar. The tradition of eating raw food has not led to any large-scale embrace of a recent food fad of eating only raw food.

Attention to detail and the practice of aesthetics on a small scale have always been among the defining, and visually the most appealing, attributes of Japan's traditional culture. Rising affluence has made many such displays more affordable as an unprecedented variety of foods and of both traditional and modern serving dishes (made of china, ceramics, glass, wood, or metal) can be used in aesthetically pleasing presentations. At the same time, this new affluence has also produced its quota of kitchen, tableware, and restaurant kitsch, and the already noted ubiquity of fast food restaurants for budget-conscious consumers has done little for upholding the best standards of Japan's admirable art of minimalist food display.

The contest between continuity and change can be also seen in the ways Japanese are eating. Continuity is everywhere on display, but rather than being preserves of a true frugal tradition, some of its forms have become major contributors to energy and environmental waste. *Hashi* (chopsticks) are a perfect example of this transformation. Modern means of mass industrial production and hygienic packaging of individual sets have created a veritable explosion of *waribashi*, disposable wooden chopsticks made from raw wood. Cheap bamboo (and also cedar and cypress) *waribashi* were introduced during the middle Edo period (when they were actually often reshaved and reused) by *sobaya*, but domestic output of disposable chopsticks rose rapidly only after World War II. Eventually nearly all of this enormous demand (now more than 95 percent of the annual use of nearly 25 billion pairs) came to be satisfied by imports, mainly from China.

Disposable boxed meals (*bentō*) have also increased in popularity as urbanization, increasing participation of women in the workforce, and a much higher frequency of rail travel—a market segment whose demand is catered to by a variety of railway *bentō* (*ekiben*), sometimes distinguished by the inclusion of local specialties (Kamekura, Watanabe, and Bosker 1989)—created a large-scale demand for throwaway varieties of this traditional meal presentation. Wooden and even ceramic containers were replaced by molded plastic, adding to Japan's considerable waste disposal problems. And given the ubiquity of fast food consumption, it is not easy to come up with inexpensive alternatives to wooden *waribashi* and plastic *bentō* boxes (with their ubiquitous plastic grass, a modern substitute for traditional bamboo grass garnish, *sasa*).

Many dietary habits have been slipping away, but some traditionally favorite, and quintessentially Japanese, foods are still consumed frequently: *mitsuba* and *konnyaku* are excellent examples of this perseverance. Where European cuisine uses parsley and Middle Eastern and Asian cuisine add cilantro to flavor soups and stews and salads, Japanese cuisine uses leaves and stalks of *mitsuba* (*Cryptotaenia japonica*), an herb virtually unknown outside Japan. Ground and extensively processed starchy root of *Amorphophallus konjac* (*konjac*, devil's tongue) yields gelatinous *konnyaku* with a high fiber (glucomannan, a water-soluble polysaccharide) content. Retailed either as small jelly-like cakes or thin white filaments (*shirataki*) packed in water, *konnyaku* can be eaten as *sashimi*, but it is usually added to hot-pot (*oden*) or simmered dishes (e.g., *shirataki* is an almost indispensable component of *sukiyaki*). And we have already noted the persistence of *nattō*.

There is also persistence in absence. Garlic has been a common and favorite ingredient in all other major Asian cuisines, notably in China, India, Thailand, and Indonesia, and the last three culinary traditions also favor liberal use of many spices, singly but more often in combinations that create effects raging from fragrant to highly spicy. In contrast, traditional Japanese cuisine had little use for garlic (*ninniku*), and it has not adopted any Asian or Western foodstuffs or meals that use it liberally. Similarly, the spice mixtures that are used in *karē raisu* are fairly mild and have little in common with their Indian counterparts (real *garam masala*).

As far as traditional high-status foods are concerned, Japanese continue to be exceptionally fond of unusual and expensive seafoods (ranging from the best *chūtoro* to *fugu*) and they remain dedicated mushroom eaters willing to pay exorbitant prices: a few perfect specimens of *matsutake* go for hundreds of dollars. But a closer look shows that some of these dietary continuities, as unique as they may be considered by many Japanese, have counterparts in other countries or regions. In China, much as in Japan, there is virtually no marine organism that would be classed as inedible, and as Chinese incomes have risen, so have the country's imports of such high-status marine foods as sea cucumber and abalone.

The Japanese fondness for mushrooms is shared in many European countries, from Russia, Ukraine, and Poland to Germany, France (wild *cepes* and *chanterelles*, cultivated *champignons*), and Italy (*porcini* and extraordinarily expensive white and black truffles). And Japan is far from being the only country with continuing horse meat consumption (viewed as an abomination in the United States and Canada). France, Belgium, Italy, Sweden, and Germany still have special butcher shops selling the sweetish-tasting meat, and there is no dietary taboo against its eating in Latin America. And eels are consumed as eagerly in China and Germany as in Japan.

Finally, the last example of continuity prevails only in comparative sense: Japan's relatively low waste of food. While in other countries we have to rely on occasional studies of household food waste or on approximate estimates derived from analyses of garbage, Japanese statistics make it easy to calculate the average per capita loss as a simple difference between food availability and actual food consumption from annual household studies. And these figures, available since 1946, make it clear that *relatively* is the key word here because in absolute terms, the recent waste of food (in energy terms, the daily mean on the order of 700 kcal/capita) has been nearly five times the level of fifty years ago (the mean in 1960 was about 150 kcal/capita). But this high loss—amounting to about 25 percent of the total daily food supply at the retail level and adding up annually to energy sufficient to feed nearly 45 million people eating 2,000 kcal a day—still compares favorably with postproduction food waste in nearly all other affluent countries.

Traditional attitudes were very different: Japanese frugality was noted during Japan's first encounter with Americans as Commodore Perry described the conclusion of a banquet:

When the dinner was over, all the Japanese guests simultaneously spread out their long folds of paper, and . . . without regard to the kind of food, made up an envelope of conglomerate eatables. . . . Nor was this the result of gluttony, or a deficiency of breeding; it was the fashion of the country. . . . The practice was universal, and they not only always followed it themselves, but insisted that their American guests, when entertained at a Japanese feast, should adopt it also. (Perry 1856, 375–376)

More than 150 years later, there are few signs of American frugality. Although many Americans may insist on taking away their uneaten portions from restaurants, America's postproduction food waste—in retail outlets, households, restaurants, hospitals, prisons, and army barracks—has reached an obscene level. Hall et al. (2009) used a model of metabolic and activity requirements to calculate the most likely food intake of the U.S. population between 1974 and 2003. Their best estimate is that it rose from about 2,100 kcal per day to nearly 2,300 kcal per day; during the same period, the average food supply rose from about 3,000 kcal per day to 3,700 kcal per day, which means that America's food waste increased from 28 percent in 1974 to about 40 percent three decades later.

A detailed survey of British food waste found that the U.K. households waste about 31 percent of purchased food (Waste & Resources Action Programme 2008), and if supermarket losses and wastes in institutional eateries and restaurants are added, the total would come close to the U.S. rate. Given the very high average per capita food supplies in all other major EU economies and the fact that (when considering typical body weights and activity levels) actual intakes in those countries cannot be higher than about 2,100 kcal a day, it is obvious that similarly high, or even slightly higher, levels of food waste (40–45 percent of the total supply) must prevail in most EU countries.

Official Japanese statistics show average per capita food intakes higher than the average supplies until 1955, an impossibility best explained by the extent of postwar black market and barter that helped to secure food that never appeared on any supply ledgers. In reality, losses must have been minimal, and even during the late 1960s, they averaged no more than 300 kcal a day or just 12 to 15 percent of the average supply. They began to grow during the late 1970s, reached a peak of about 750 kcal a day by 2000, and have been declining slightly ever since, although they remain at just over 700 kcal a day. Waste composition analysis shows average daily food loss amounting to nearly 500 grams per capita, with half of the total generated by households (and with about 40 percent of that loss potentially edible) and the rest by industrial food processing, stores, and restaurants.

Fruits, vegetables, and seafood have the highest household waste ratios, and a closer look shows that leftovers (so-called plate waste) are not significantly different among various age groups. However, direct disposal (throwing away uncooked or spoiled food or opened items past their expiration date) is higher among people twenty years old and younger, as well as among people over age fifty; the reason appears to be that younger people do not plan their purchases well and older people tend to buy too much (Ministry of Environment 2006). Various steps to recycle these wastes as animal feed, composts, or feedstock for methane generation intensified after the adoption of new rules about waste recycling that came into effect in 2001. Yet another sign of changing attitudes has been the recent appearance of Japanese polypropylene doggy bags that look like boxes that bakeries use to package take-home cakes and that can withstand temperatures up to 70°C.

Reverse Flows of Foodways

Before World War II the only notable influence of Japanese cuisine was to be found in Japan's colonies at the time, Taiwan and South Korea. Given the rapid postwar growth of Japan's international economic, social, and cultural interactions, it was only a matter of time before some of the country's unique foodways found their ways abroad. There were always small Japanese restaurants, drinking establishments (*izakaya*), and food stores in Hawaii and in North American cities with relatively large concentrations of Japanese immigrants—above all in Honolulu, San Francisco, Vancouver, and Los Angeles—but it took several decades before Japanese food (or its American adaptations) diffused beyond major cities.

The first successful post–World War II Japanese restaurant chain outside Japan was Benihana, a *teppanyaki* steakhouse. Wrestler Hiroaki (Rocky) Aoki (he died in 2008) opened his first tiny New York restaurant in 1964, and the concept became a success. Now a Miami-based and NASDAQ-listed company, Benihana has eighty franchises on four continents, and the restaurants now serve not only a variety of steaks but also tuna, shrimp, lobster, and salmon, as well as tofu steaks and a variety of *sashimi* and sushi (Benihana 2010). Benihana's early success stemmed not only from its meaty meals but also from its theatrical food presentation with chefs working with large knives at a *teppanyaki* table in front of the diners.

The first important component of the Japanese cuisine that came to wider public attention in the United States was bean curd. Its ascendance was part of a new social trend that began during the late 1960s and was a product of the baby boom generation's coming of age. The rise of environmental consciousness, interest in vegetarian diets, and admiration of Buddhism by many young Americans provided a perfect combination for embracing tofu as a symbol of better eating. When Shurtleff and Aoyagi published *The Book of Tofu* in 1975, they were convinced that the world was facing a serious food crisis, predicted that within ten or twenty years (i.e., no later than by 1995) the origins of U.S. dietary protein would be reversed (with 80 percent coming from plant foods), and believed that new tofu shops in America "will make an invaluable contribution to the betterment of life on our planet during the years ahead" (Shurtleff and Aoyagi 1975, 13).

The realities turned out to be very different: there has been no real global food crisis, animal foods still supply about 65 percent of America's dietary protein, and a small number of America's artisanal tofu shops have not made any noticeable difference to America's diet. In fact, even in Tokyo, the number of such small shops fell below a thousand by 2008, with four or five of them going out of business every month. Tofu made by larger producers eventually made it into a wider distribution after the 1980s, and a few brands, as well as a variety of tofu-based meat substitutes, are carried by all major U.S. supermarket chains. Nevertheless, annual per capita consumption remains minuscule, rising higher only among vegetarians, who make up no more than 3 percent of American population.

No other foodstuffs are seen as more quintessential components of the Japanese diet than rice and seafood, both combined in various kinds of sushi, undoubtedly the most successful Japanese culinary export (Watanabe 2004). Specialized sushi restaurants began to open in Los Angeles during the 1960s, and one of these, Tokyo Kaikan, set up by EIWA group, made culinary history as its chef, Ichirō Mashita, tried to cater to non-Japanese tastes by substituting buttery avocado for *toro* and combining it with crabmeat and cucumber to create a new *makizushi*, now the world-famous California roll (Issenberg 2007). An inside-out arrangement (with rice sometimes covered with *tobiko*) and the use of imitation crabmeat came later. Hirotaka Matsumoto opened the first specialized *sushiya* in Manhattan in 1975 (Matsumoto 2006), and sushi restaurants ranging from genuine ones to poor imitations subsequently spread to all major cities in North America and Australia.

Some of the more expensive sushi restaurants were both very traditional and innovative, none more so than Manhattan's Nobu, which Nobuyuki Matsuhisa opened in 1994. It offers sushi influenced by the chef's Latin American experience, including such signature morsels as *tiradito* (sashimi-like fish slices dressed with juice dominated by lime and chili peppers), yellowtail with jalapeño, and bonito with *chimichurri* (an Argentinian hot sauce made with parsley, garlic, oil, vinegar, and red pepper). Nobu's New 2009 New Year's Eve *omakase* offered signature choices as well as lobster sashimi with foie gras and miso-marinated foie gras for $150 to $200 per person (Nobu 2009). Nobu became one of the celebrity magnets in the city, and its success led to the eventual opening of an upmarket chain of Nobu restaurants in other countries.

In contrast, inexpensive American establishments have based their business on serving *makizushi* varieties that are not found in Japan. Fashioned to American tastes and expectations, these rolls are usually larger than their Japanese counterparts, the rice (*sumeshi*) is sweeter, and the fillings are usually composed of several colorful ingredients, not just a single kind, as in the traditional *tekka-* and *kappa-maki*. In addition to the now ubiquitous California roll, other notable creations include the New York roll, with sliced apple, avocado, and salmon; the Philadelphia roll, with smoked salmon, cream cheese, and cucumber; the Texas roll, with cooked beef and cucumber; the spider roll, with crab, avocado, and spicy mayonnaise; and the caterpillar roll, with crabmeat and cucumber on the inside and avocado and *unagi* on the outside. There are also egg salad rolls with hard-cooked eggs and mayonnaise, holiday rolls with turkey and cranberry salsa, and assorted vegetarian rolls (usually with thinly slivered cucumbers and carrots or with lettuce or mushrooms).

This American, or fusion, sushi has made it back to Japan, but it remains uncommon: California roll has yet to become a common offering, for example. Sushi is now a truly worldwide phenomenon: it can be ordered in the food courts at large shopping malls throughout North America, as well in the most expensive hotels in Australia, China, and

Brazil, and small sushi restaurants can be found in America's heartland in Oklahoma and Kansas as well as on the Rive Gauche in Paris (Issenberg 2007; Matsumoto 2008). Some of it is authentic, lots of it incorporates local taste preferences (in Mexico, it is dipped into spiced sauces, and in the United States, it gets slathered with flavored mayonnaise). And these restaurants also serve other Japanese dishes—always *miso shiru* and almost always *tempura* and *teriyaki*. And the conveyor-belt sushi (*kaiten-zushi*, first introduced in Japan in Osaka in 1958 and now available in thousands of restaurants around Japan, with individual portions placed on a conveyor for customers' selection) has also made it abroad with many popular sushi restaurants.

There are no reliable figures about the total number of restaurants that serve Japanese food abroad, but in 2007 the Ministry of Agriculture, Forestry and Fisheries put the total at 20,000 to 25,000 and increasing rapidly. This total was cited in a draft document that proposed voluntary participation in a program run by Japan's government to recommend foreign restaurants serving Japanese foods once they meet assorted criteria regarding ingredients, Japanese culinary skills, sanitary practices, and the overall restaurant atmosphere, tableware, and menu (Ministry of Agriculture, Forestry and Fisheries 2007). This global sponsorship, managed by a private Japanese outfit with government support, has not found enthusiastic acceptance in the entrepreneurial world of restaurant food service.

The worldwide diffusion of *rāmen* has been already noted: no other foodstuff originating in Japan has enjoyed such worldwide diffusion as instant noodles, dried or in a cup: they are now eaten around the world. This leaves only one additional Japanese dietary habit that has seen a major diffusion abroad: avid drinking of green tea, a rarity twenty years ago. In some ways, this is a misleading attribution, because the overwhelming majority of green tea that is now offered by every major Western tea company—mass marketers as Lipton and Tetley, upmarket brands such as Kusmi and Mariage Frères, and wellness promoters as Celestial Seasonings and Tazo—has little in common with the real Japanese *sencha*. They are closer in appearance and taste to various Chinese green teas. The driving force behind this diffusion (which now also includes green tea–based soft drinks) is the claim about the tea's disease-preventive and curative powers.

This section would not be complete without noting a common food-related product with Japanese commercial origins: monosodium glutamate (MSG), a sodium salt of glutamic acid. The acid is naturally present in many foods, above all in seaweeds, cheeses, soy and fish sauces, and tomato, and by 1907 Japanese chemist Kikunae Ikeda had identified the glutamate as the source of the fifth basic taste, which he called *umami* (Kawamura and Kare 1987; Yamaguchi and Ninomiya 2000). He patented the isolation of the compound from *konbu* in 1908, and its commercial production began soon after under a trademark name *aji no moto* (essence of taste) by an eponymous company. Ajinomoto eventually expanded its operations worldwide (it has been in the United States since 1956), and it produces the compound by fermenting sugars (Ajinomoto 2010).

MSG has become one of the world's most commonly used food additives and the leading flavor enhancer. Even if it is not identified exactly on a product's list of ingredients, it may be contained in "seasonings" or "hydrolyzed protein." Ingestion of relatively large amounts of MSG has been credited with such (transitive) postprandial effects as numbness at the back of the neck, general weakness, palpitations (Kwok 1968), and other effects (including asthma), soon ascribed to what became known as Chinese restaurant syndrome caused by liberal use of MSG in Chinese restaurant cooking (Raiten, Talbot, and Fisher 1995). These concerns have persisted despite the fact that double-blind placebo-controlled studies have shown no evidence of any discomfort in general (Geha et al. 2000) and no MSG-induced asthma (even in history-positive subjects) in particular (Stevenson 2000).

This closes our systematic examination of dietary trends, changes, and continuities that have marked Japan's dietary transition since the beginning of the twentieth century and particularly since the mid-1950s. Now we will turn to what we see as the most important consequences of these dietary shifts: their possible effects on longevity and health, and their environmental impacts. The former links are notoriously difficult to demonstrate in unequivocal terms, while the latter effects—ranging from changing land use, demand for water, large-scale interference in nitrogen cycle due to intensive fertilization and alteration of marine food webs—can be illustrated with indisputable findings.

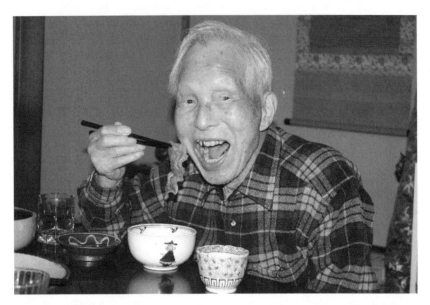

Japan has a relatively higher percentage of centenarians than any other modern affluent country. Diet must play a role in this achievement. Here Katsunori Kishida, born in May 1911, enjoys eating meat (Niko Kishida).

4
Diets and Well-being: Health and Longevity

For many individuals, their genetic inheritance or excessive environmental exposure is the most important factor determining their health and longevity. For the poorest traditional populations, it was impossible to rank their inadequate diets, their dismal living condition, and their extraordinarily hard labor as the most important factors of their poor health and shortened life expectancy. But today nutrition is undoubtedly the principal external factor in maintaining a disease-free quality of life and prolonging a healthy and active life span for large populations that live in (what must be considered in a long-term historical perspective) excellent accommodations, benefit from reasonably well-controlled exposure to environmental pollutants and toxins, have access to preventive medical care and timely treatment of diseases, and have relegated hard labor to machines.

In Japan's case, this link between diet and health and longevity seems to be particularly worthy of a closer look because two generations ago the country rose to the top of the global life expectancy ranking for both males and females and has kept that position ever since. Add to this the relatively low frequencies of several major diseases (cardiovascular morbidity and several major cancers, including those of breast and prostate), contrast these realities with well-known stresses of Japan's urban living (crowded housing, long commutes and working hours, short vacations), and what emerges is an intriguing possibility that the Japanese diet is a key factor in suppressing disease and prolonging life. We will look first at some key specific foodstuffs and beverages whose regular intake have been identified as important contributors to Japan's outstanding longevity. Then we appraise the general health benefits of the Japanese diet—

above all, the country's relatively modest (and actually declining) overall food energy intake.

Searching for Dietary Clues to Longevity

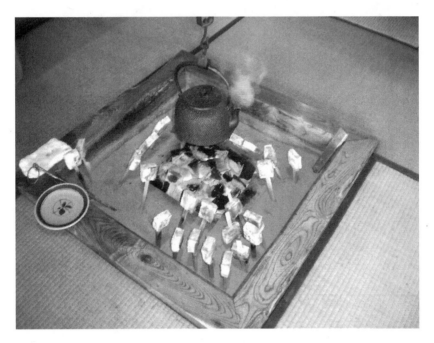

Figure 4.1
An essential ingredient of a frugal and healthy Japanese diet: bean curd (tofu) toasted in an old-fashioned hearth in a small rural inn. No other country consumes as much tofu per capita as Japan does. (V. Smil)

Few links are apparently as self-evident, but in reality as complex and as contentious, as those between nutrition and health, or more specifically between intakes of food energy and individual macro- and micronutrients on one hand and the prevalence of various diseases and frequency of incapacitating morbidity and average longevity on the other. The link is most obvious and the consequences are unmistakable in extreme situations, either with chronically inadequate food energy and protein intakes due to repeated harvest failures or to largely man-made famines. In today's world, the case of serious malnutrition is perhaps best exemplified by recurrent food shortages in the arid, conflict-beset Horn of Africa. And even the twentieth century had no shortages of major famines, with the largest two in India's Bengal in 1943 (Uppal 1984; Weigold 1999) and between 1959 and 1961 in China, the world's worst famine caused by delusionary Maoist policies.

The first victims of recurring food shortages are prematurely dying infants and people who are already ill, followed by emaciation of the general population and an exodus of refugees seeking food aid. During the twentieth century, a number of famines caused the deaths of more than 1 million people in a matter of months, and China's great famine of 1959–1961 killed more than 30 million people (Smil 1999). Tokugawa Japan had three major famines: the Kyōhō famine of 1732, the Tenmei famine of 1783–1787, and the Tenpō famine of 1833–1837. The last was the most widespread of the three events as it affected not only cold northern areas but extended to the middle of Honshū (Jannetta 1992; Nakamura 2000). There is no agreement on the human toll of these famines. The Tenpō famine was the last such event in Japan's history: all of the twentieth-century food shortages were managed by food rationing and, in the case of the most serious supply shortfall in 1945 and 1947, timely American food deliveries.

Nevertheless, decades of only adequate food energy supplies and sub-optimal protein intakes were unmistakably reflected in shorter stature and lower body weight, as well as in the health, morbidity, and life expectancy of affected populations. In this sense Japan of the first half of the twentieth century represented only a more pronounced version of a situation that could be encountered in many other countries that were still in transition from traditional, largely rural to modern, largely urban societies. Stunted growth has been the most common result of a limited availability of food, and although stunting conveys a sense of permanent damage, the prevalence of shorter and lighter bodies (even now widely encountered around the world) is not incompatible with good health and a decent life expectancy. A little-appreciated fact is that even in Europe, most people born before 1950 matured without expressing fully their growth potential, and as a result their children are much taller than they are.

Shorter stature and lighter weight are successful adaptations to reduced food availability, and Japanese anthropometric, mortality, and life expectancy statistics are an excellent confirmation of the fact that this adaptation works well for a population that is forced to cope with a less-than-optimal though far from crippling food supply. The Japanese experience is thus yet another example of a phenomenon that has been appreciated since the 1980s: some populations can use their food more efficiently even when their intake is appreciably below standard expectations, and with rates as much as 20 to 30 percent below the predictions based on metabolic studies of European populations (Garby 1990; Kanade, Gokhale, and Rao 2001).

Japanese Life Expectancy

Japan's historical statistics (some of them available for more than 100 years) also demonstrate the benefits of improving nutrition, and none of these impacts is as impressive as the country's record longevity. Increased life expectancy at birth is obviously an outcome of a complex interaction of several interlinked processes, with nutritional improvements being a very important, but not necessarily the dominant, factor. Other important correlates of increased life expectancy range from rising per capita gross domestic product (GDP) or family income, improving housing conditions and typical educational attainment to general satisfaction with life, good public sanitation, widely available preventive health care, and accessible and effective medical treatment. But after considering all of these critical factors, a case can be made that the increase in the average longevity of the Japanese population has been significantly correlated with the nation's diet.

This case is strengthened by the fact that an international comparison of key variables shows Japan's solid achievements but no exceptional record on any of those accounts. In 1985–1986, when Japan's life expectancy at birth became the world's longest (surpassing that of Iceland) the country's per capita GDP, as well as average family income, were well below the U.S., French, and Swedish levels, particularly when the comparison is done in terms of purchasing power parities. Japan's housing has been a target of foreign and domestic criticism, including during the 1980s, when the country enjoyed an otherwise uncritical admiration during its seemingly unstoppable economic ascent to what was to be an unchallenged global primacy. Japan's compulsory education produces a highly literate population, but the country's postsecondary institutions are not exceptional, and their overall record is not superior to the norm of those in Western countries.

Public opinion polls gauging level of happiness (or satisfaction with life) show the Japanese being perennially among the less satisfied people within the group of affluent nations (World Database of Happiness 2009): on a scale of 0 to 10, their scores have been mostly between 5.5 and 6.0, much like those in Italy, and much lower than, for example, in France (most commonly around 7.5) and the United States (where the scores have been fluctuating between 7.2 and 7.8). Japan has some admirable traditions of initiatives that make for good public health, ranging from the provision of clean water in Japan's large cities to personal cleanliness, with a frequency of regular bathing that surpassed the contemporaneous preindustrial Western norms (Hanley 1997). But it also has a more recent, and unenviable, record of lagging sewer installations—by 1985 nearly a third of Japan's urban population was not connected to sewers, and the nationwide rate was only 67 percent as recently as 2005 (Statistics Bureau 2011b)—and environmental pollution. All in all, the country has been hardly a paragon of progressive sanitation.

And as for the overall level of health care, Japan does not spend an unusually high share of its GDP on health care—recently, about 8 percent compared to more than 9 percent in Sweden, 10 percent in Canada, and 11 percent in France (Organization for Economic Cooperation and Development 2009)—and there are no widely used comparative indicators of basic medical services (such as the number of doctors, nurses, and hospital beds per 1,000 people) that would set the country apart from or well above other affluent countries with universal medical insurance. Consequently, these findings of good but far from exceptional levels for other key determinants of longevity strengthen the claim for a significant role that nutrition plays. And this claim is bolstered by the timing of Japan's highest longevity gains since 1950.

In 1900 Japan's average life expectancy at birth was just short of 43 years for males and just over 44 years for females, putting Japan at a very similar level with Italy (about 43 years for both sexes) and behind France (45 and nearly 49 years) and significantly behind the United States (48 and 51 years) and Sweden, where the expectancy was 53 years for males and 55 years for females (Kinsella 1992). By 1950 the Japanese means increased to, respectively, nearly 60 and just over 63 years, gains of about seventeen and nineteen years. For comparison, Italian male expectancy lengthened by nearly twenty-one years for males and twenty-four years for females during the same period (to nearly 64 and just over 67 years), the French gains were over eighteen and nearly twenty-one years (to nearly 64 and more than 69 years), and the American longevities increased by almost eighteen and nearly twenty-one years (to 66 and almost 72 years). Consequently, Japan's pre-1950 performance lagged behind the gains of the richest Western countries.

In contrast, during the second half of the twentieth century Japan has outdistanced all of these countries with gains of nearly 12 years in male life expectancy and an astonishing 22.6 years in average female longevity (United Nations 2009; graph 4.1). The country's population moved to the first place on the global longevity list in 1985 for females and a year later for males, and it has held those positions ever since. Between 2000 and 2005, Japan's life expectancies of 78.3 and 85.7 years were well ahead of both the U.S. (75.8 and 80.6 years) and French averages (75.8 and 83.1 years). Attributing these indisputable achievements to particular components of the Japanese diet is a counterproductive task: even if diet were the sole determinant of longevity (which is not the case), its impact is a result of a lifelong, complex interaction of individual nutrients, numerous metabolically active compounds, and overall levels of food intakes.

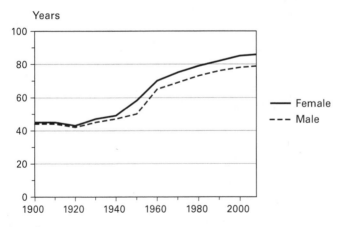

Graph 4.1
Mean life expectancy at birth for Japanese females and males, 1900–2008.

Seafood, Soy Foods, and Green Tea

Given the reductionist propensity of modern science, it is not at all surprising that a great deal of attention has been devoted to several unique
attributes of Japanese diet, above all to its unparalleled consumption of
seafood, its relatively high intake of soybean-based foods, and its ubiquitous drinking of green tea. Before highlighting some important results
of these studies (ranging from statistically significant confirmation, to
intriguing suggestions, to clear findings of no discernible links), it is
necessary to stress that as all other epidemiological findings, they are not
proofs of causal relationships but merely of quantifiable statistical associations or their absence.

Beneficial health effects of fish consumption have been attributed
primarily to relatively high concentrations of two omega-3 polyunsaturated fatty acids, eicosapentaenoic acid, and docosahexaenoic acid. Herbivorous species accumulate these acids directly from feeding on plankton;
carnivorous species secure them by predation. Higher intake of omega-3
fatty acids has been associated with reduced inflammation (due to the
increased production of prostaglandins that inhibit the inflammatory
process), lower low-density lipoprotein (LDL) cholesterol levels, and low
incidence of ischemic heart disease. So far the most comprehensive examination of fish consumption and mortality from all causes, ischemic heart
disease and stroke (it examined data from thirty-six countries and ten
time periods between 1961 and 1991), found that reduced mortality risk
was associated with fish intake in all of those instances (Zhang et al.
1999). This association remained statistically significant even after the
two countries with by far the highest fish consumption (Iceland and
Japan) were excluded from the analysis.

An interesting Japanese study contrasted the diets of two village
populations, a fishing village and a farming village in Mie prefecture,
and the prevalence of atherosclerotic disease (Yamada et al. 2000).
Adults in the fishing villages, who consumed 1.6 to 1.8 times more fish
than in the farming village, had higher serum levels of ωomega3 fatty
acids and strikingly fewer plaques in their carotid arteries—only about
5 percent compared to 66 percent for males and less than 8 percent
compared to nearly 52 percent for females. But the study did not find
that higher intake of fish and higher serum levels of omega-3 fatty

acids were associated with lower levels of plasma fibrinogen which was identified by other studies as an independent predictor of cardiovascular disease (CVD).

A cohort study supports the hypothesis that high fish consumption may reduce the risk of fatal prostate cancer (Truong-Ming et al. 2009), while data from the Ohsaki National Health Insurance Cohort Study (ONHICS), which was initiated in 1994 among more than 40,000 healthy adults between forty and seventy-nine years who had no history of stroke, coronary heart disease, or cancer at its start, revealed no association between fish consumption and the risk of colorectal cancer (Sugawara et al. 2009). And while Yamagishi et al. (2008) confirmed an inverse association between fish and omega-3 fatty acid intakes and heart failure, they found that associations with heart attacks were statistically insignificant and were absent with mortality from all strokes and from cardiac arrest.

It is also necessary to consider possible negative effects of higher intakes of fish, particularly carnivorous species (tunas, swordfish, sharks) at the top of their respective food chains, due to their relatively high levels of methylmercury (Endo et al. 2005). Frequent consumption of seafood also increases the intake of dioxins, highly toxic polychlorinated environmental pollutants that tend to concentrate in food lipids. A study in Tokyo found that dioxins consumed in fish and shellfish make up more than 50 percent of the total daily load, with the intake of polychlorinated biphenyls having the highest rate of increase (Sasamoto et al. 2006). Whale meat has also high levels of mercury as well excessively high levels of polychlorinated biphenyls and organochlorine pesticides (Simmonds et al. 2002).

Central nervous system effects of ingesting methylmercury are well documented, ranging from paresthesias (prickling and tingling in the extremities), muscle weakness, unsteady gait, and impaired vision, hearing, taste, and smell all the way to memory loss (Sanfeliu et al. 2003). Minamata disease, caused by bioaccumulation of mercury released by Chisso Corporation, was perhaps the most tragic demonstration of these effects (Tsubaki and Takahashi 1986). Although there is no such danger following regular consumption of a variety of fish species, concerns remain about cumulative effects of consuming fish with elevated methylmercury level, particularly by pregnant women.

No other modern country comes close to Japan's average consumption of soy-based foods, and the intakes are even higher among older adults. In terms of soy protein, they vary between 6 and 11 grams per day, which translates to 25 to milligrams per day of isoflavones, the bioactive components whose possible health benefits have received a great amount of research and public attention (Messina, Nagata, and Wu 2006). Isoflavones (the three major groups present in soybeans are genistein, daidzein, and glycitein) are heterocyclic phenols, also known as phytoestrogens because they are structurally similar to the hormone and bind to estrogen receptors (Isanga and Zhang 2008). Other bioactive compounds present in soybeans are saponins, phytic acids, and phytosterols.

Health benefit claims made on behalf of regular consumption of soy foods range from their antiatheroslerotic activity and reduced risk of coronary heart disease (mainly due to the lowering of serum cholesterol) to bone loss prevention and lower incidence of breast, prostate, intestine, liver, stomach, and skin cancers. They have been also promoted as a safer alternative to hormone replacement therapy for postmenopausal women and as meat and dairy substitutes. At the same time, soybeans (like other legumes) contain various antinutritive factors, including those that interfere with the absorption of nutrients in the small intestine.

A closer look shows many uncertainties stemming from these studies. Some of the recent epidemiological work confirms certain long-standing claims. For example, a prospective cohort study of soy product intake and stomach cancer death found a significant inverse association when comparing the highest and the lowest daily consumption in adult men (Nagata et al. 2002), and Nagata et al. (2007) credited soy isoflavones with a significantly decreased risk of prostate cancer (most likely due to their weak estrogenic activity). Kokubo et al. (2007) found that high isoflavone intake was associated with a reduced risk of both cerebral and myocardial infarctions in Japanese women, particularly after menopause, and Nagata et al. (2001) identified a strong inverse association between the consumption of soy products and hot flashes.

But recent studies of lipid-lowering activity of soybeans have come up with inconsistent results, and assessments of isoflavone benefits in preventing CVD, postmenopausal bone loss, diabetes, and some cancers remain inconclusive (Sacks et al. 2006; Xiao 2008), and a prospective study suggested that consumption of soy foods has no protective effects against breast cancer (Nishio et al. 2007). Moreover, potentially adverse effects of antinutritive factors present in all soy-based foods are still only poorly understood, and in the case of prostate cancer, Nagata et al. (2007) concluded that because of higher phytoestrogen levels in Japanese diets (and hence higher serum concentrations), the results may not be used as the basis for soyfood-based preventive intervention in other populations.

As for the third unique attribute of the Japanese diet that has been linked to some impressive health benefits, both in vitro studies and animal experiments have confirmed that the beneficial effects of green tea must be ascribed to catechins. These are polyphenolic flavonoids whose mass may constitute as much as 40 percent of the dry weight of tea leaves. In general, the antioxidant effects of polyphenolic compounds in foods and drinks are expected to provide some chemoprevention (with in vitro studies showing inhibition of cancer cell growth) or to have disease-modifying effects (Halliwell 2007). But actual claims that can be made on the basis of longer-term epidemiological studies are relatively modest. After scores of epidemiological studies, the evidence is fairly clear: specific health benefits of frequent green tea drinking remain unclear.

The most comprehensive review of clinical evidence of the benefits of regular drinking of green tea concluded that the observational studies are inconclusive as far as the prevention of most cancers is concerned (Clement 2009). A large prospective study of nearly 20,000 Japanese men found no evidence of beneficial effects in the prevention of prostate cancer (Kikuchi et al. 2006) or reducing the risk of stomach cancer among males (Hoshiyama et al. 2004). However, those studies suggest that habitual drinking of green tea may protect against hypertension and may reduce the risk of stroke, a finding best supported by the results of the ONHICS (Kuriyama et al. 2006). That study also found an inverse association between green tea drinking and mortality due to all causes but no effect on cancers. In contrast to this, Inoue et al. (2009) followed more than 200,000 adults for a decade and found that green tea drinking may decrease the risk of one type of gastric cancer in women, but had no effect on another type of gastric cancer in either women or men.

More surprising, interventional studies have shown reduced relapses of colorectal adenomas following their resection, as well as increased survival rates for women with epithelial ovarian cancer. Shortly after Clement (2009) published his review, a new report, also based on the ONHICS, indicated that daily drinking of five or more cups of green tea compared with less than one cup a day was associated with a lower risk of hematologic malignancies (Naganuma et al. 2009). And yet another recently concluded investigation based on the ONHICS looked into the effects of catechins against infectious agents (demonstrated in vitro and in animal experiments) and found that green tea consumption was associated with a lower risk of death from pneumonia among women (Watanabe et al. 2009). But perhaps the most intriguing recent finding (given the aging of many affluent populations) is that more frequent drinking of green tea was associated with a lower prevalence of depressive symptoms among elderly Japanese seventy years and older (Niu et al. 2009).

But this too may be less meaningful than it seems. Tsubono et al. (1997) discovered that consumption of green tea by Japanese men is significantly associated with intakes of ten other kinds of foods and four key nutrients. The strongest links are with the frequent eating of vegetables, soy foods, fruits, and seaweed, and also with dairy products and eggs. Tea drinkers also had lower intakes of lipids, and their drinking may thus be just a marker of diets that could modify the risks of CVD and some cancers. Moreover, Fukushima et al. (2009) found that coffee is the most important source of polyphenols in a modern Japanese diet, supplying 50 percent of the total compared to 34 percent for green tea and 48 percent for all teas.

Japanese Diet and Health

Given the complex, dynamic, and aggregative nature of any association between health and nutrition, it might be more sensible to ascribe any effects on longevity and any health benefits of the Japanese diet to its totality rather than to keep singling out some of its outstanding

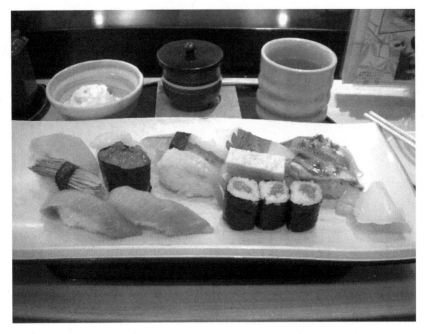

Figure 4.2
A common component of Japan's remarkably restricted food energy intake, perhaps the most likely reason for the country's record longevity: a simple sushi meal (photographed in one of Tokyo's famous *sushiya* in the precincts of the Tsukiji fish market) that provides a combination of protein and carbohydrate with a minimum of fat. (V. Smil)

components. This inquiry must first address an important distinguishing attribute of the Japanese diet: the effect of the traditionally high intake of salt on mortality and life expectancy. Although it is easy to agree that the traditional intakes were so high that they had to have a number of negative effects, more recent consumption of salt presents a puzzle: although it has declined from its postwar highs, the average intake is still too high, and it is generally seen as detrimental—and yet it has not prevented steady declines of diseases associated with elevated salt consumption and has not affected the nationwide increase in life expectancy.

The second general characteristic of the Japanese diet is a relatively low consumption of lipids in general and saturated animal fats (eaten separately as butter or in meat) in particular. This dietary feature should have a highly beneficial impact on the incidence of several diseases associated with increased consumption of lipids and cholesterol, above all on the incidence of coronary heart disease (CHD). And yet this too presents a puzzle as far as health effects are concerned because CVDs associated with the consumption of these fats have been steadily declining even as the consumption of lipids has been increasing. The third defining characteristic of modern Japanese diet is a close match between average intakes and expected food energy needs.

The low incidence of chronic overeating combined with level of physical activity that still exceeds the typical North American norm is well reflected in very low rates of obesity. Japan's National Health and Nutrition survey classifies adult obesity as body mass index higher than 25, and in 2006 29.7 percent of males older than twenty years and 21.4 percent of females in the same age category were above that limit (Ministry of Health, Labour, and Welfare 2009). In contrast, the international definition of adult obesity is a body mass index higher than 30 (BMI above 25 is classed as overweight); accordingly, the Japanese adult obesity rate was still only 3.9 percent in 2005 when the U.S. rate had surpassed 33 percent (the highest prevalence among the leading economies) and the European shares ranged from 10 percent in Italy to about 23 percent in England (National Obesity Observatory 2009). Once again, this contrast is also a puzzle because a closer look at the best available data concerning actual average food intakes does not indicate commensurately higher levels of chronic overeating outside Japan.

High Salt Intakes

High salt intakes have been identified (thanks to a combination of experimental, epidemiological, and intervention studies) as one of the key factors helping to explain (because of its effect on hypertension) higher risks of CVD in general and stroke in particular (Strazzullo et al. 2009). These risks are especially high in societies where the intake has been well above the recommended level, which is as low as 3 grams a day in Canada and 4 to 5 grams a day in the United States. In some prefectures, traditional Japanese diets contained as much as 20 to 25 grams of salt every day (Sakata and Moriyama 1990). Annual nutritional survey data are available for salt only since 1973, and they document stable intakes for the next two decades, with a mean of 13.3 grams per day during the late 1970s and 12.9 grams per day during the late 1990s.

And yet during the same period of time, age-adjusted mortality due to cerebrovascular events had declined quite impressively from about 350 per 100,000 in males and 240 per 100,000 for females to, respectively, only about 75 and 45 per 100,000, and the decline has continued ever since with the 2007 rates at about 55 and 32 per100,000 (National Cancer Center 2009). Moreover, these rates are not starkly different from the U.S. rates. In 1975 the Japanese age-adjusted stroke mortality for males was twice as high as for white U.S. males and about 60 percent higher for females; by 2005 the Japanese male mortality was only 38 percent higher and the female mortality was 20 percent lower (National Institutes of Health 2009) even though the average U.S. salt intake is less than one-third of the Japanese rate. There is clearly more to this trend than a simple inverse salt intake–stroke mortality explanation.

Some components of Japanese diets may have a protective effect. Epidemiological studies have found that mortality from cerebrovascular events (stroke, intracerebral hemorrhage, cerebral infarction) was inversely associated with an intake of green and yellow vegetables and fruits (Nagura et al. 2009; Takachi et al. 2008; Sauvaget et al. 2003a). However, Nakamura et al. (2008) found that high fruit and vegetable intake was associated with only a modest reduction of CVD risk in women but not in men. Similarly, in a large (nearly 40,000 adults) cohort in Takayama, there was an inverse association between adherence to a diet recommended by the Japanese food guide (with its high intake of vegetables and fruit) and CVD (as well as non-CVD and noncancer mortality) among women but no statistically significant link between the adherence score and reduced mortality was found among men (Oba et al. 2009).

And while the Hiroshima/Nagasaki Life Span Study found a significant inverse link between fruit consumption and stroke (daily intake resulting in 35 percent reduction of the risk in men and 25 percent in women), it also found that intake of animal foods, including eggs, dairy products, and fish, may also be protective against intracerebral hemorrhage (Sauvaget et al. 2003b). That finding is clearly linked to intakes of dietary calcium, which have doubled from the traditionally low rates of the dairy-free Japanese diet of about 270 milligrams per day in 1950 to 550 milligrams per day in 2000, and an inverse link of higher calcium intakes with stroke was confirmed by a large prospective study that followed more than 41,000 Japanese adults for more than a decade (Umesawa et al. 2009).

An additional puzzle about the effects of salt on disease is presented by Japan's trend in stomach cancer. High salt intakes have been linked with a high incidence of stomach cancer in Japan, and several studies have indicated that environmental factors are more important in explaining that high stomach cancer incidence and mortality than the congenital ones (Hirohata and Kono 1997; Matsuzaka et al. 2007). But the age-adjusted stomach cancer mortality has been steadily decreasing even as salt intakes have stabilized at a still fairly high level: for males the rates fell from nearly 80 per 100,000 in the early 1960s to about 40 per 100,000, but they are are still two to three times higher than in other affluent countries where salt intakes are lower than in Japan (National Cancer Center 2009).

Again, other factors are at play, including still undesirably high salt intake, and high prevalence of heavy smoking (Matsuzaka et al. 2007). On the other hand, higher consumption of green and yellow vegetables and fresh fruit may have preventive effects. Curiously, a study that showed a Western breakfast to be inversely associated with stomach cancer risk also found that the consumption of high-salt foods (*miso shiru, tsukemono*) is not significantly associated with the stomach cancer mortality in both sexes (Tokui et al. 2005). Obviously declining mortalities due to both stroke and stomach cancer cannot be explained by a simple association with a single micronutrient.

Low Consumption of Lipids

Even after several decades of Westernization, the average intake of fats and oils accounts for no more than a quarter of all food energy in a typical Japanese diet, significantly below the means of nearly all other affluent nations where lipids supply a third or more of the total. Is this exceptional overall leanness of the Japanese cuisine the most important variable that could be used to explain the beneficial effects of the prevailing diet on healthy aging and a record longevity? There was a time when the epidemiological consensus would have been affirmative.

A very low-fat diet contains no more than 15 percent of food energy in fat: 33 grams for an average daily intake of 2,000 kcal (Lichtenstein and Van Horn 1998). The preindustrial Japanese diet was clearly in that category, and lipid intakes remained low in many rural settings for many years after World War II. Beneficial effects of exceptionally low shares of lipids in the Japanese diet first received major international attention when Noboru Kimura included two Japanese cohorts (the farming village of Tanushimura and the predominantly fishing village of Ushibuka) in the famous Seven Countries Study that investigated the links between CHD and lifestyle factors, particularly dietary fat intake (Keys 1970; Seven Countries Study 2009).

The study involved sixteen cohorts of men aged forty to fifty-nine in seven countries, and its baseline surveys were done between 1958 and 1964. The results showed a strong positive association between the average intake of saturated fats and CHD mortality. Not surprisingly, men in the two Japanese locations had the lowest age-standardized twenty-five-year CHD mortality, respectively 30 and 36 per 1,000 compared to rates in excess of 100 per 1,000 in the United States and northern European cohorts and 40 to 90 per 1,000 in the Mediterranean cohorts; only a Crete cohort had lower mortality, at 25 per 1,000 (Menotti et al. 1999). Multivariate analysis showed that consumption of butter, lard, margarine, and meat were the most significant predictors of mortality, and higher intakes of legumes, oils, and alcohol had the strongest negative correlations. But the Seven Countries Study did not include any cohorts from France, and hence it missed the French paradox: a high intake of saturated fat and dietary cholesterol coexisting with low CHD mortality (Renaud and de Lorgeril 1992).

This paradox extends to other parts of Mediterranean Europe (Masia et al. 1999), and the explanation of the phenomenon now goes beyond the originally suggested primary factor of frequent drinking of red wine and embraces a diet rich in fruits and vegetables, complex behavior concerning wine drinking, and regular physical activity (Ferrières 2004). And a later follow-up of the Seven Countries Study uncovered the Japanese paradox: between 1958 and 1989, typical per capita consumption of fats, meat, and dairy products increased, as did the mean cholesterol level, average body mass, blood pressure, and the percentage of overweight men—but CHD mortality did not change (Toshima, Koga, and Blackburn 1994).

These findings now extend to the 1990s as comparisons between U.S white men and Japanese men showed similar cholesterol levels and similar systolic and diastolic pressures (differences in risk factors were more overweight in the United States, more smoking in Japan) but the U.S. CHD mortality about twice the Japanese rate (Sekikawa et al. 2003). And a prospective study with a seven-year follow-up by Shimazu et al. (2007) confirmed that despite its relation to high sodium intake and hypertension, the Japanese diet was associated with a lower risk of CVD mortality. Yet again, focusing on individual dietary factors fails to explain that substantial difference. Nor is there any clear agreement about the cardioprotective components of the Japanese diet. High vegetable consumption is suggested as a major factor, but Takachi et al. (2008) concluded that only a higher consumption of fruit, and not vegetables, was associated with a significant lowering of CVD mortality and that neither fruit nor vegetable consumption made any difference in the risk of total cancer.

In concluding this section on the beneficial effects of diet and longevity, it might be illuminating to note the importance of yet another factor that has nothing to do with nutrition: Japanese call it *ikigai*, life worth living, and *raison d'être* is perhaps the closest rendering in a European language. Satisfaction in life comes only to those who have it naturally or those who work hard to uncover it. Sone et al. (2008) used the data from the ONHICS to calculate hazard ratios for the all-cause and cause-specific mortality according to different *ikigai* categories: individuals who did not have a strong sense of *ikigai* had an increased risk of all-cause mortality specifically attributable to CVD and external causes but not to cancer.

Japanese Diet and Caloric Restriction

In view of the uncertainties and contradictory findings regarding the links between health and longevity, on one hand, and specific foodstuffs or major diet characteristics, on the other, an argument can be made that the dietary composition or some general features of typical

Japanese food intakes may be actually of a secondary consideration and that the overall modest level of daily food energy intake is the factor that provides the greatest benefits. This conclusion rests on what are now well-documented effects of caloric (or dietary) restriction on extending life spans of organisms. Discovery of this link goes back to experiments with rats at Cornell University during the 1930s (McCay, Crowell, and Maynard 1935), and the key requirement is to realize that that effect can be achieved only when an adequate level of all nutrients is combined with a significantly reduced energy intake (hence the term CRON—calorie restriction with optimum nutrition), and that restrictions of specific nutrients without an overall reduction of food energy intake have no such effect.

Even those early rodent studies showed that the extension of an average life span was due to the postponed onset of major illnesses (including some cancers), reduced blood pressure, faster glucose metabolism, and enhanced immune response. Subsequent extensive experiments proved that in laboratory settings, restricted diets delay the onset of age-related illnesses and prolong life spans for a diverse range of organisms: from protozoa and invertebrates (spiders, water fleas, ticks, cockroaches, molluscs) to fish and mammals, particularly to rodents (Weindruch and Walford 1988; Sohal and Weindruch 1996). These findings led to an obvious question: Would caloric restriction work as well in humans?

Wilcox et al. (2006, 173) concluded that caloric restriction "not only *will* work but in fact available epidemiological evidence indicates that CR *may already have* contributed to an extension of average and maximum lifespan." Their conclusion was based on the diet-longevity link in Okinawa where the aging cohort (sixty-five years and older) clearly exhibits the caloric restriction phenotype with associated extension of longevity as well as with relatively low disability rates in advanced age. Ryūkyū cuisine is an obvious hybrid of Chinese, Southeast Asian, and Japanese foodways: sweet potato was traditionally the dominant carbohydrate staple (supplying up to 70 percent of all food energy), and the everyday diet included a variety of vegetables and seaweed combined with *tōfu*, and relatively small amounts of fish and even smaller amounts of pork; pickled vegetables and fruits were nearly absent.

Those elderly Okinawans subsisted on a low-calorie diet for decades—in 1950, when the average Japanese food intake amounted to 2,068 kcal and 68 grams of protein per day, the two averages were merely 1,785 kcal and 39 grams in Okinawa—and their overall food energy intake was about 11 percent below the level that would normally be expected given their body mass and activity level (Sho 2001; Wilcox et al. 2007). Yet by 1955 Okinawan longevity surpassed the Japanese mean, and by the beginning of the twenty-first century, the difference (averaged for both sexes) was about 1.5 years when compared to the average and 3.8 years compared to the maximum (99th percentile) Japanese life span.

Again, uncertainties abound. Other specific factors, or their combinations, might be responsible, ranging from a lower glycemic index of dominant carbohydrates (sweet potatoes in Okinawa versus rice in Japan) and high levels of energy expenditures required by traditional farming methods to genetic differences and psychosocial peculiarities. But perhaps the best conclusion is that the long-lasting caloric restriction has made the difference but that the actual longevity gain has been relatively small (an order of magnitude less than has been observed in mice), exactly as expected when taking into account evolutionary considerations, reproductive investment, and differences between rodents and humans in the reaction norm connecting longevity to food energy intake (Phelan and Rose 2005, 2006).

In addition, Speakman and Hambly (2007) remind us that conclusions from animal studies involving optimal (and pathogen-free) environments and little physical exertion by the experimental subjects are not applicable to human populations exposed to infections and required to earn a living. They also stress that if the restriction of food energy intake begins in one's forties, the eventual benefits will be small, and turning to such a diet during one's sixties may not add any years to life expectancy. The full effect of energy-restricted diets might be realized only with lifelong (or nearly so) deprivation, a most unlikely prospect for contemporary Japan where childhood obesity has been increasing.

At the same time, it is interesting to speculate to what extent the average Japanese, and even more so the typical Okinawan, longevity was affected by a temporary but prolonged period of mild caloric restriction (mostly 5 to 10 percent below the expected norm) during the first postwar decade. Japanese anthropometric data show that neither males nor females surpassed their previous maxima of average body weights (52.9 kg for sixteen-year-old males in 1941, 48.6 kg for sixteen-year-old-females in 1944) until 1956. Phelan and Rose (2006) found the increase in the upper bounds of longevity attributable to caloric restriction to be as low as 2.1 percent and as high as 6.8 percent, that is, between one and a half and more than five years, the range that corresponds to the actual differences between longevities in Japan and other affluent nations.

Japanese food supply has been more than adequate for half a century, and it is obvious that no caloric restriction has been practiced. At the same time, recent annual surveys of actual food intake report averages below 2,000 kcal a day, and so it would be interesting to know how close these rates are to intakes that would be expected by taking into account the specific metabolic and activity rates of the Japanese population and its sex and age distribution. The latter shares are readily available from demographic statistics and the latest dietary reference intakes that have been published (Ministry of Health, Labour, and Welfare 2004) can be used to calculate Japan's expected food energy consumption: its mean, with moderate activity, comes to about 2,100 kcal a day, and it is approximately 1,800 kcal a day when assuming light physical activity as the norm.

In today's Japan, with its largely sedentary occupations and an aging population, the most likely value is somewhere between these two rates. Simply splitting the difference gives about 1,950 kcal day, whereas the latest surveys indicate actual food energy intake very close to 1,900 kcal per day. This means that on the average, Japan's population is consuming just about as much energy as is expected on the basis of its sex and age distribution and its typical activity level. No deliberate population-wide caloric restriction is taking place, but there is also no sign of any population-wide overconsumption. The mean intake may actually come a few percent below the expected level, but the uncertainties of such accounts also mean that the match could be almost perfect. This remarkable reality confers considerable health benefits because the absence of any population-wide overeating along with maintenance of appropriate body weights reduce the frequency or postpone the onset of common age- and diet-related illnesses—and it also remains a key indicator of continuity amid the changes brought by Japan's dietary transition.

In the next chapter, we turn to a quantitative assessment of the environmental impact of this dietary transition. This inquiry is complicated by Japan's high post-1960 dependence on food imports, which means that we have to examine not only land, water, and fertilizer needs (and impacts) of Japanese agriculture but also the input requirements and environmental impacts of all imported commodities used for food or feed. Similarly, in the case of seafood, we have to look beyond catches by Japanese fleets and beyond domestic mariculture in order and assess the impact that Japan's demand for fish and shellfish has on the oceans.

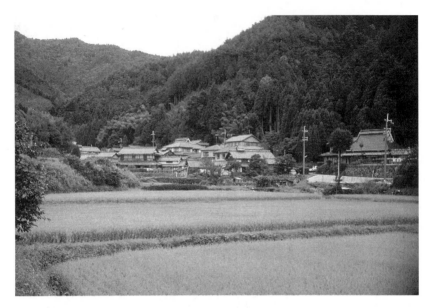

Rice fields, villages, and mountains, Japan's typical agricultural landscape north of Kyoto. (V. Smil)

5
Environmental Impacts: Land, Water, Nitrogen, and Ocean

Agriculture is a clever manipulation of artificial ecosystems in order to maximize their net primary productivity. Some of these agroecosystems are relatively species rich, involving complex rotations of crops, even interplanting, as well as the maintenance of perennial plants in hedgerows or tree groves separating the fields, contributing biodiversity and reducing soil erosion. Other agroecosystems are brutally simplified monocultures, with continuous plantings of a single crop, usually a staple cereal. All of them share the same essential requirements for land, water, macronutrients, and micronutrients; all of them would have their yields lowered by excessive competition from weeds; and most of them may need protection from microbial attacks and grazing by insects and vertebrates.

This means that productive agroecosystems require suitable soil (or considerable, and often continuous, efforts to improve soil quality by enhancing its organic matter), a reliable water supply, timely provision of nutrients (the need dominated by supplies of nitrogen, almost always the most important macronutrient whose timely delivery determines the final crop yield), and services that will keep both weeds and heterotrophic invaders in check. In traditional agroecosystems, these essential services were delivered by a great deal of human exertion, sometimes made easier by using animals or simple mechanical devices. As a result, large amounts of labor were needed for field preparation (plowing, harrowing), construction of irrigation infrastructures, collection and application of organic fertilizers, and weeding.

In modern agroecosystems, these services make use of fossil fuels or electricity to power field machinery (including irrigation pumps), transport inputs to fields and harvests to markets, and indirectly to produce all agricultural machinery, synthesize agricultural chemicals (fertilizers, herbicides, fungicides, pesticides), and process crops by drying, milling, extraction, or fermentation. Rising inputs of fuels and electricity have changed the human role in agriculture from that of a critical prime mover of the system to a controller and manipulator of direct and embedded energy flows and, of course, an indispensable developer of better cultivars and more productive ways of cropping. Fisheries and mariculture have also become highly dependent on external energy inputs of fuel and electricity, and in affluent countries, more energy is used in food processing, storage, wholesale, and retailing than in agriculture and fishing.

Environmental impacts of modern food production and food supply systems are thus both universal and country specific. The most commonly encountered problems in cropping are losses of arable land due to the encroachment of residential and industrial construction and transportation networks, degradation of soil quality (most often due to poorly controlled soil erosion and declining content of organic matter), unsustainable water withdrawals and wasteful water use in irrigation (processes leading to depletion of aquifers and, in arid regions, soil salinization), and excessive applications of nitrogenous fertilizers leading to impacts ranging from elevated emissions of nitrous oxide to eutrophication of fresh and coastal waters.

Japan, thanks to its high share of bunded paddy fields, does not have a severe soil erosion problem, and during the past generation, its losses of arable land to nonagricultural uses have been less important than the voluntary abandonment of farmland, a consequence of shrinking domestic cropping and increasing food imports. As far as water use is concerned, monsoonal Japan has an abundant supply, and its well-managed irrigation systems use it quite efficiently. Nevertheless, intensive fertilization required to produce high yields from limited farmland has burdened Japanese waters with excessive nitrate loads and put arable land at the top of major sources of a greenhouse gas: nitrous oxide (N_2O) from nitrification and denitrification of nitrogenous fertilizers. Rice paddies are the second largest source, after ruminants, of another greenhouse gas: methane (CH_4) generated by anaerobic fermentation in anoxic soils. And Japan's exceptionally high consumption of seafood has a large impact on the status of major fish stocks and the maintenance of marine biodiversity.

Moreover, modern energy-intensive agriculture has also made comparative production advantages more pronounced, a development has been furthered by the fact that the intercontinental food trade became much more affordable as a result of inexpensive commodity shipments (dry, wet, frozen) in large bulk carriers and containerized exports of processed food. Japan's high reliance on food imports, with most of them coming not from nearby Asian countries but other continents, thus creates additional carbon dioxide (CO_2) emissions from transportation. Quantifying these impacts is not easy because the additional costs due to transportation and environmental changes, for example, might be partly, or even entirely, offset by lower production costs in exporting regions that enjoy considerable comparative advantage in natural resources.

Land

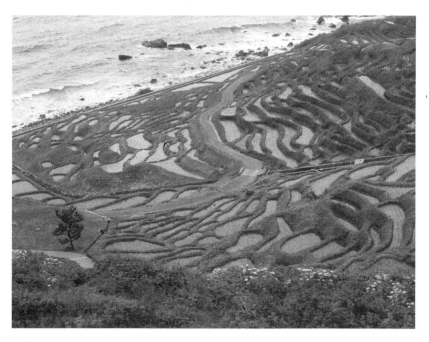

Figure 5.1
A scarcity of land led to intensive cropping, including elaborate terracing. (K. Kobayashi)

Land Requirements

Data on aggregate totals of all agricultural land (subsuming all arable land and area under permanent, usually tree, crops) are the ones that are most readily available over extended periods of time, but even if a country did not engage in any agricultural trade, it may not be the best choice for quantifying the land requirements of its food and feed production because it could include considerable areas devoted to industrial crops, a category that ranges from fiber crops (cotton, flax, hemp) and tobacco to sericulture that requires extensive mulberry plantings. Fortunately, Japan (in its historical statistics series) has long-term agricultural land use data disaggregated by major crops (starting in 1878 for cereals, legumes, and sweet potatoes, with the series almost complete for all other major crops since the first decade of the twentieth century), so it is easy to make the necessary adjustment by subtracting the areas devoted to industrial crops.

Only in a country that produced all of its food domestically and with no or few agricultural exports would a reliable data series on planted (or, better yet, harvested) areas of all major crops be the only information needed to quantify long-term changes in annual land requirements for food and feed harvests. This was essentially true as far as Japan's food supply in 1900 was concerned. After a brief period of rice exports (around 3 percent of total rice harvest) during the late 1880s (Ōmameuda 2007), food imports began to rise beyond a negligible level during the 1920s, and by the late 1930s, shipments of rice and sugar supplied notable shares of overall domestic demand. This trend of rising dependence on foreign purchases of food was restarted during postwar reconstruction, and it acquired an entirely new component as Japan became a major importer of not just essential foodstuffs (above all, wheat and soybeans) but also a leading buyer of feedstuffs (above all, corn and soybeans) destined for domestic production of poultry and red meat. By the end of the twentieth century, Japan had also become a major importer of meat and a notable buyer of other animal products.

Consequently, any meaningful quantification of land requirements for Japan's food supply must add all foreign agricultural land used to produce imported food and feed crops, as well as the land that was used to produce feed crops in the countries that are Japan's major suppliers of meat and other animal foods, to the changing totals of land used for domestic production of food and feed crops. Accounting for the land requirements in food-exporting countries is a challenging task, particularly in the case of meat exports. But at least there is no need to take care of reverse flows: Japan's agricultural exports (dominated by apple exports to Taiwan) never reached levels high enough to make any real difference to overall domestic land use needs. Indeed, inevitable error margins entailed in quantifying the foreign land use needs are substantially larger than the land totals claimed by Japan's minuscule plant food exports.

Japan's Agricultural Land

Japan's mountainous and often steeply sloping terrain has been always the most significant physical limit on the expansion of the country's agricultural land, and during the twentieth century, the combination of a nearly tripled population and large-scale industrialization and urbanization claimed large areas of flat and potentially cultivable land for houses, factories, and transportation corridors. Early in the twentieth century, modernization of Japanese farming eased this fundamental limitation primarily by achieving some remarkable improvements in productivity, most notably of its already high rice yields. More recently the country's food supply became steadily more dependent on food and feed imports, and as a result, the total cultivated area has declined to the lowest level in modern history.

At the beginning of the twentieth century, Japan had about 5.25 million hectares (Mha) of cultivated land, and the total was almost identical in 1990. During the intervening decades, the cultivated area rose first, reaching a peak of about 6.05 Mha in 1921; by 1929 it was down to 5.85 Mha, and by 1937 it was once again back to 6.05 Mha. Another decline took place during and right after the war, with the total getting as low as 5.05 Mha in 1950. After a decade of expansion, Japan's cultivated area reached its greatest-ever extent in 1961, with 6.086 Mha. Subsequently it has declined every year, down to 4.6 Mha in 2009 (table 5.1; graph 5.1). Most of these shifts are explained by the changing area of paddy fields, which expanded from about 2.7 Mha in 1900 to the record size of 3.4 Mha in 1969—but by 2009, it was barely above 2.5 Mha.

Table 5.1
Land for domestic production and food and feed imports, 1900–2005

Year	Cultivated area (Mha)	Land for imported		Total land claim (Mha)	Per capita land claim (m²/capita)	Foreign share (percent)
		Crops (Mha)	Animal foods (Mha)			
1900	5.2	0.2	—	5.4	1,200	4
1925	5.9	1.4	—	7.3	1,200	20
1935	5.9	2.1	—	8.0	1,150	25
1950	5.0	1.7	—	6.7	800	25
1955	5.0	3.0	—	8.0	900	37
1975	5.5	9.5	0.8	15.8	1,400	65
2000	4.8	11.0	3.0	18.8	1,500	74
2005	4.7	10.5	3.0	18.2	1,425	74

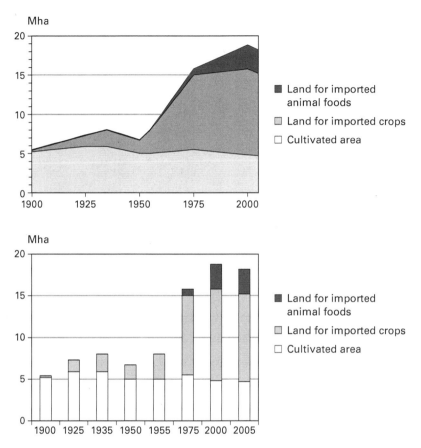

Graph 5.1
Land area required for domestic production and imports of food and feed, 1900–2005.

When comparing the changes of the total cultivated area during the twentieth century, Japan's decline of about 8 percent is less than the pullbacks for France (about 17 percent) and Sweden (at about 22 percent), but when measuring the Japanese decline from the peak level of 1961, the change, at 20 percent, is very similar. But the Japanese loss of agricultural land is greater than in the United Kingdom (where the total area was down just 2 percent), while both of the world's two largest economies, the United States and China, cultivated significantly more land in 2000 than they did in 1900—China about 15 percent more and the United States 26 percent more (Smil 2001). But these comparisons tell only part of the story because unlike during the preceding centuries, when crop yields remained stagnant or increased only slowly, the twentieth century saw some impressive productivity gains, and Japan was at the forefront of these improvements.

Soybeans were the only major crop whose average yield did not at least double during the twentieth century, but it came close, with a nearly 90 percent increase. Rice yields grew 2.4 times, slightly more than those of sweet potatoes, wheat yields tripled, and potato yields more than quadrupled. But even these impressive gains produced only modest increases in the overall output of major annual crops (cereal, tubers, and legumes). In 2000 their total phytomass (harvested parts and crop residues) was only about 1.3 times the 1900 level, while during the same period, the British harvest of these crops had tripled, the French output grew 3.6 times, and the U.S. production of total cereal, tuber, and leguminous phytomass grew 4.1-fold (Smil 2001).

Moreover, most of the gain in Japan's primary agricultural productivity took place early in the century: overall output of the three major crop categories had expanded considerably between 1900 and 1925 (total phytomass increased 1.5 times), it remained fairly stable until the early 1950s, rose slightly during the next three decades, and has since seen a substantial decline. Declining intensity of cultivation has been reflected by the country's falling multicropping index (the sequential number of crops cultivated in a given field in one year): in 1900 it averaged about 1.33, by 1950 it was around 1.25, and in 2000 there was, at least statistically, no multicropping as the index slipped below 1.0 (0.95). Not surprisingly, this trend has been accompanied by a much higher production of grass for feed: its annual harvest increased more than ten times between 1960 and the year 2000.

International comparisons with other populous and densely inhabited nations show how limited Japan's arable land is. In 2007 it prorated to about 0.034 hectares per capita (340 m^2, that is, a square of 18.5 by 18.5 meters), just marginally higher than the South Korean mean (0.033 hectares per capita) but only about a half of the Vietnamese average. The Indonesian mean is more than two and a half times times greater, China has nearly three times as much arable land per capita as does Japan (so does the United Kingdom), and the multiples for Germany, France, and the United States are, respectively, about 4, 8.5, and 16 (Food and Agriculture Organization 2011b). If this limited availability of arable land were the only constraint on the country's food production, could Japan feed itself solely by domestic harvests? This, of course, is a loaded question and the answer depends on first answering another key question: Feed itself at what level?

At the beginning of the twentieth century, Japan produced virtually all of its overwhelmingly vegetarian diet (supplemented by a small amount of seafood protein) from domestic crop cultivation. For most of the 1890s, it was actually a small net exporter of rice (maximum of 125,000 tonnes in1894), and in 1900 it imported about 1.8 percent of its total rice consumption. Between 1898 and 1902, the country's self-sufficiency ratio was 97 percent for unmilled rice, 100 percent for barley, and 92 percent for wheat (Ogura 1980). After adding a small amount of sugar imported from its new colony of Taiwan, Japan's overall food self-sufficiency ratio was close to 97 percent in 1900. This means that the Japanese agriculture needed about 5.4 Mha, or 1,200 m^2/capita of farmland to feed nearly 44 million people in 1900, with less than 4 percent of the land outside the country. With today's considerably higher yields, much less land should be required to produce the same overwhelmingly vegetarian diet—but the country's population nearly tripled during the twentieth century.

Even when assuming that the current share of food energy derived from seafood would not change and that all postharvest food losses were kept to minimum, the country would need to produce at least 2,300 kcal a day (as opposed to 2,100 kcal a day in 1900, an inadequate amount resulting in widespread stunted growth). An unrealistic assumption determines the bottom: if the Japanese were willing to eat a diet composed of only brown rice (60 percent of all food energy), sweet potatoes, and soybeans (each supplying 20 percent of food energy), they could grow, with the current yields, 2,300 kcal a day from about 550 m^2 of arable land per capita. With the current farmland of less than 5 million-hectares, this could feed nearly 85 million people, but when we assume the historical maximum of about 6 Mha, it could feed about 110 million people.

A more nutritious but still basically vegetarian diet would need at least 700 m^2/capita, a balanced diet supplying 2,300 kcal a day (with about 15 percent from animal foodstuffs) would need around 1,000 m^2/capita, and a diet with 25 percent of food energy coming from animal foods could require no more than 1,500 m^2 if dairy products, rather than meat, supplied most of the animal protein. These calculations make it clear that even with today's high average crop yields, Japan does not have enough farmland to feed itself even at the Bangladeshi level (1,900 kcal/capita). Any adequate diet thus requires considerable imports, and the current diet with 15 percent of all food energy coming from animal foodstuffs (excluding seafood, frugal in comparison with the means prevailing in North America and the EU) means that no other modern economy has to depend as much on food imports as Japan does because of its land constraints.

Land for Rising Crop Imports

At the beginning of the twentieth century, Japan's small food imports, dominated by rice, wheat, and sugar, were all for direct consumption or processing by food industries. This pattern prevailed until after World War II, when imports of animal feedstuffs began to rise and eventually dominate Japan's crop imports. At the same time, its food imports began to diversify, and by 1975, only rice, potatoes, and vegetables were of solely or overwhelmingly domestic cultivation. Calculations of Japan's requirements for foreign agricultural land are made easier by the fact that the country's imports of field crops and crop-derived commodities have always been dominated by only a few items—above all, feed corn, soybeans, and oil seeds—whose cultivation takes place in a small number of countries. Unavoidable errors inherent in quantifying the land demands of these key commodities are greater than the area totals for many minor crop imports.

These uncertainties arise largely because it is impossible to apply highly accurate yield averages to individual export commodities. Even if all the imports of a particular crop were to come from a single country, the quantification of the amount of agricultural land needed for these imports in producing countries might not be just a simple matter of dividing the relevant import total by corresponding average yield. This procedure would yield accurate totals in the case of a small producer with no or minimal regional variation of yields—but it could create a significant bias in the case of such large exporters of foodstuffs as the United States or Brazil.

Perhaps the most obvious example is that of the U.S. corn exports to Japan: average nationwide yield of the crop is significantly lower than the productivity in the two most important corn belt states, Iowa and Illinois (which are also the primary contributors to the country's corn exports). Because international trade statistics do not provide any subnational attributes, we must calculate overall land requirements with an important caveat that some of those figures most likely are overestimates of actual needs because any substantial exports usually come from the most productive agricultural regions. But in order to be as accurate as possible, we have not used any common approximations and have chosen instead appropriate national (U.S., Canadian, Brazilian) crop yields for specific periods. This complicates the calculations but improves their accuracy.

Because of a high degree of multicropping (and intercropping), this approach is much too difficult to apply in the case of imported vegetables, where some generic approximations must be used. Comprehensive data needed for these calculations for the pre–World War II period are available from the Food and Agriculture Organization's (FAO) precursor, the International Institute of Agriculture (IIA), also headquartered in Rome (IIA 1926, 1937), while the postwar trade statistics are more readily accessible in both official Japanese and FAO's (2011c) databases.

While in 1900, Japan was virtually (about 97 percent) self-sufficient in producing a basically adequate but suboptimal diet, by 1925 the country was becoming a significant importer of rice, wheat, and sugar. Net imports of rice, mostly from Japan's two colonies, Korea and Taiwan, amounted to nearly 16 percent of the total supply. Imported wheat accounted for nearly 40 percent of the total supply, and about 380,000 tonnes of sugar were brought from Taiwan. Other imports exceeding 10,000 tonnes were rapeseed, soybeans, and sesame seeds (IIA 1926).

Average crop yields in the principal exporting countries were used to calculate the total extent of arable land required by Japan's food imports in 1925. This claim was dominated by rice with about 670,000 hectares; wheat imports added 470,000 hectares, sugarcane needed to produce the imported sugar occupied about 125,000 hectares, and the total for soybeans and oilseeds was about 110,000 hectares, for a grand total of close to 1.4 Mha. At that time, Japan's cultivated land was just over 6 Mha, and industrial crops (fibers and tobacco) accounted for only about 2 percent of that total. This means that food production for Japan's nearly 60 million people required about 7.3 Mha in 1925, or almost exactly 1,200 m²/capita, a rate nearly identical with that of a quarter-century earlier, but with almost 20 percent of the overall land burden shifted overseas. This pattern changed little during the last prewar decade.

In 1935, Japan's rice imports from its two colonies were almost 17 percent of the overall supply (Hayami and Ruttan 1970). The country also imported about 85 percent of its sugar supply from Taiwan and 60 percent of all soybeans, mostly from the occupied Manchuria, and about 200,000 tonnes of various oilseeds (mostly rapeseed and cottonseed). But continued imports of wheat were largely offset by substantial exports of wheat flour (IIA 1937; FAO 1959). Assuming appropriate average yields that prevailed during the mid-1930s, the total land requirements for Japan's crop imports were 2.1 Mha (table 5.1). With the domestic crop area of 5.9 Mha, the grand total of 8 Mha means that the average diet in the mid-1930s required about 1,150 m²/capita, with 25 percent of the burden shifted overseas. Given the inherent uncertainties of these calculations, the two rates should be seen as identical at about 1,200 m²/capita. In 1925 the country imported about 13 percent of globally traded rice, and its imports of wheat and sugar each accounted for only about 3 percent of the respective totals. In 1935 it imported about 25 percent of all traded rice and 9 percent of all traded sugar.

Land for Postwar Food Imports
Japan's food supply in 1950, five years after the end of World War II, was inferior to that of the late 1930s. Limited food imports could not make up for lasting shortfalls of domestic production: rice and sugar imports were a fraction of the peak rates reached during the late 1930s, only the imports (a large part of them gifts) of American wheat and wheat flour were significantly above the prewar maxima (the average for the years 1948 to 1952 was about 1.6 Mt of grain equivalent), and there were still no significant imports of meat or processed meat products. Following the same procedure used for the prewar calculations of land claimed by Japan's food imports, we put the total area needed to grow the foreign crops at about 1.7 Mha. When added to the domestic crop-

land of 5 Mha this means that only about 800 m^2 of farmland were used to produce what amounted to an obviously inadequate average food supply. But then the situation began to change rapidly, with plant food imports sharply up by 1955—but still with no significant meat imports.

In 1954 Japan's recovering economy had finally surpassed its highest prewar gross domestic product. A year later it had its record rice harvest (at 12.4 Mt, nearly 30 percent above the previous year), soybean harvest was up by an even higher margin (nearly 35 percent), and rising incomes allowed higher food purchases and more diverse imports. Nearly all of the imports that became important during the 1930s (rice, wheat, soybeans, sugar) were significantly up compared to 1950, and a new import pattern was emerging as the country was buying, for the first time in its history, substantial quantities of foreign feedstuffs in order to boost its output of animal foodstuffs. In 1955 imports of U.S. corn surpassed 300,000 tonnes; they were supplemented by more than 100,000 tonnes of sorghum, and an increasing share of soybean imports went for feeding—but virtually no scarce foreign exchange was allocated to imports of animal foods.

Arable land needed to cultivate Japan's 1955 imports of grain crops, oilseeds, and sugar added up to at least 3 Mha, and the domestically cultivated area was, at just above 5 Mha, still below its prewar peak; the total of 8 Mha prorated to about 900 m^2 per hectare, about 12 percent above the 1950 level—but because of a relatively high population growth (6 million people were added in just five years), this had translated into only a marginal improvement of actual per capita food intakes. Food supply had stabilized and began to expand, but the real improvements were yet to come. They began as a combination of a temporary expansion of cultivated land (from 5.14 Mha in 1955 to more than 6 Mha until 1965), higher domestic crop yields, and rising imports of feed crops for expanding domestic meat and dairy production. By 1965 the total meat output was nearly four times the 1955 level, and by 1975 it was two and a half times as large as a decade earlier, while milk output had quintupled between 1955 and 1975.

Not surprisingly, American crops have dominated Japan's feed imports. Feed corn became the country's most important import during the late 1960s, when it surpassed imports of wheat destined for direct food consumption. Total annual imports have been around 16 Mt since the mid-1980s, with the U.S. share fairly steady at about 95 percent. In 2000, Japan bought directly more than 6 percent of America's corn crop (and it imported more of it indirectly in U.S animal foods). That imported crop required about 1.8 Mha, an equivalent of nearly 40 percent of Japan's arable land, or roughly all of the land planted in corn in South Dakota.

By the century's end, wheat (the United States, Canada, and Australia have been its main suppliers) remained Japan's second largest grain import, and it was the world's largest wheat importer, with only less than 10 percent of the imported total going for animal feed. In contrast, the use of barley, traditionally the third most important grain import, is about equally split between food and feed uses, and sorghum (mostly from the United States), the number four grain import, has been for feeding only. In total, by the century's end, Japanese food and feed grain imports reached 27 Mt, by far the largest in the world and accounting almost exactly for 10 percent of the global cereal trade (South Korea, with less than 13 Mt was second, and China and Egypt had each bought less than 10 Mt). Little had changed during the first decade of the twenty-first century, with Japan buying just over 9 percent of all traded cereals in 2005.

In addition to its top position in cereal trade, Japan is also a major buyer of soybeans and other oilseeds. In the year 2000, its soybean imports (equal to about 10 percent of all world exports) were second only to China's; by 2005 its share was down to about 6 percent. Once again, there is a high degree of dependence on the United States. Imports of American soybeans began in 1946 with a small shipment of less than 3,500 tonnes, all of it for food. A decade later, Japan became the largest importer of U.S. soybeans, a position it has held ever since (Brazil is now a distant second). Japanese soybean imports from the United States surpassed 1 Mt in 1960 and the peak was reached in 1983 with 4.6 Mt; in aggregate, between 1946 and 2010, the United States exported about 160 Mt of soybeans to Japan, and about 85 percent of all soybeans consumed in Japan in fifty years since the mid-1950s came from the United States (Conlon 2009a).

In 2000, when Japan imported about 3.6 Mt of U.S. soybeans, their yield averaged about 2.5 tonnes per hectare: this means that some 1.4 Mha of U.S. farmland were devoted to these exports, and equivalent to about 30 percent of Japan's total cultivated area in that year. By 2005 somewhat lower imports and higher U.S. yields reduced the area to about 1.1 Mha. Rapeseed has dominated the imports of other oilseeds, with Canada as its traditional main supplier. Sesame imports are a distant second in the oilseed category. During the last two decades of the twentieth century, falling domestic production, rising incomes, and gradual internationalization of tastes also brought higher imports of fruits and vegetables, as well as more wine, coffee, cocoa, and nuts.

Detailed trade and agricultural statistics for the postwar decades make it easy to identify the principal exporters of all major plant foods imported by Japan, apply appropriate yields, and calculate the changing claims that the Japanese dietary transition has put on foreign farmland. This claim tripled between 1955 and 1975 when it surpassed 9 Mha, and by 2000, it stood at 11 Mha. That total was more than twice as large as all of Japan's arable land (4.8 Mha in the year 2000), and it was an area almost equal to that of all farmland in Germany (11.8 Mha). But since the 1970s, Japan's claim on foreign arable land has had to consider yet another element: its imports of animal foodstuffs.

For decades, Japan's protectionist measures kept its domestic meat and dairy market closed to imports (Longworth 1983; Conlon 2009b). Until the late 1970s, the United States, now the principal supplier of meat to Japan, exported annually less than 10,000 tonnes per year of beef and a similarly insignificant amount of pork. Liberalization of food trade led to multiplication of Japan's meat imports, from about 0.7 Mt in 1985 to almost 2.8 Mt by the year 2000. This made Japan the world's largest buyer of meat, accounting for more than 11 percent of the world trade. Subsequently imports stabilized and then marginally declined. In 2000 beef was the single largest meat import (just over 1 Mt) with pork close behind. But by 2005, the ranking was sharply reversed, with twice as much pork (nearly 1.3 Mt), largely a result of import bans on U.S. beef in December 2003 due to concerns about bovine spongiform encephalopathy, which was discovered in September 2001 in Japanese cattle (Becker 2005). Imports of chicken have fluctuated mostly between 0.6 and 0.7 Mt year since the mid-1990s, while the imports of dairy products rose from 2.2 Mt in 1990 to nearly 4 Mt in 2000.

Accounting for agricultural land used to produce imported animal foods is a much more complicated matter than calculating the land claims of Japan's crop imports. The challenge is made easier by the fact that the United States, the principal supplier of Japan's imported meat, has excellent information regarding feed requirements for the production of all animal foodstuffs and that these statistics have been available since the first decade of the twentieth century (U.S. Bureau of the Census 1975; U.S. Department of Agriculture 2008). The data series on feed consumed per head per unit of production converts all inputs to grain corn equivalents, its output is the live weight of animals or unit weight of milk and eggs, and it shows gradual improvements of feeding efficiency in some cases and stagnation in others. In 1975 it took about 1.1 kg of feed to produce 1 kg of milk, and by the year 2000, that ratio was down to 0.73. The rates for broilers (around 2.3) and pigs (between 5.5 and 6.0) showed little change, and (as expected given their large mass and long time to reach slaughter weight) beef production remains by far the most inefficient way of producing meat, with ratios of feed to live weight averaging around 12.

These ratios can be easily recalculated in terms of carcass weight or edible weight (most meat is exported as chilled carcasses or as specific lean or fatty cuts) by using typical average conversion rates (Smil 2000). But it is not possible to use these ratios as simple multipliers in order to calculate the requisite amount of feed and, hence, the overall areas of cropland needed to feed the animals. Such a simplification would work only if the animals consumed just corn or some fairly uniform diets composed of a few major plant species. In reality, modern feeding practices rely on a wide variety of concentrate feeds, wastes, and roughages.

Concentrate feed includes grains (in the United States, dominated by corn and including sorghum, barley, and wheat), legumes (soybeans and beans), by-products of grain milling and oil pressing (above all, brans, oil meals, and cakes), and livestock products (inedible fats, blood and bone meals, dried milk, fish oils and meals), and urea. Many kinds of waste organic matter are often fed to pigs, and roughage (from grazing or from consuming hay and silage) must supply a large portion of cattle rations. All arable land used to produce concentrate feeds as well as planted forages (mostly leguminous cover crops such as alfalfa and clover) must be included when calculating farmland claims. Other forages (above all, cereal straw) and all crop by-products and animal and fish feeds can be ignored in this land claim calculation because the farmland needed to produce them has been already accounted for in the crop harvest or no land is needed for their supply. Because these comparisons are limited to claims on arable land, we make no attempt to calculate the amount of grazing land (pasture) needed to produce the beef and dairy products that Japan imports.

Perhaps the most realistic approach to quantifying the land requirements of Japan's animal food imports, and one that is supported by good data series, is to use the U.S. information in order to find the average yield of America's animal food protein per unit of land planted to concentrate and forage feed crops (U.S. Department of Agriculture 2008). In 1975 it was about 125 kg per hectare, and by 2000, it rose to about 200 kg per hectare, mainly as a result of higher corn yields. Japanese animal food imports rose from nearly 1.5 Mt in 1975 to 6.8 Mt in 2000 or, in terms of animal protein, from about 100,000 to just over 600,000 tonnes. The import-to-yield quotient should give a good approximation of overall farmland requirements: about 800,000 hectares in 1975 and 3 Mha in the year 2000.

Arguments against this approach include an obvious fact that not all animal products imported to Japan originate in the United States and that feeding practices in other countries may differ substantially from the U.S. norm. Fortunately, a closer look dispels this concern. Canada has been the leading supplier of pork, and Canadian producers follow the same rearing practices as their American counterparts. But because Canadian barley, a commonly used pig feed in Canada, and corn yields are lower than in the United States, the use of the American mean will somewhat underestimate the land requirement in Canada. Similarly, chicken imported from China, Thailand, and Brazil (recently the three leading suppliers) is produced by the same intensive concentrate feeding in confinement as in the United States, while the yields of concentrate feeds produced in those countries are generally lower than in the United States. As for beef, more of Australia's cattle (in 2000 most of Japan's beef imports came from the United States and Australia) is now fed, much as it is in the United States, with concentrates in feedlots before slaughter.

Using an American average is likely to overestimate the overall farmland need only in the case of dairy foodstuffs, the source of about one-fifth of Japan's imported animal protein. This is because most of Japan's dairy imports (dominated by cheese, and including much smaller amounts of butter and dried milk) have been coming from Australia and New

Zealand, where dairy production is largely pasture based, with supplementary concentrate feeding. But in this instance, even a 20 percent error would translate to a shift smaller than 5 percent of the grand aggregate; moreover, two alternative calculation methods have resulted in similar results of between 2.5 and 3.5 Mha for the year 2000, and there is another excellent confirmation of this range by a larger study of water and nitrogen flows in the international trade of pork and chicken (Galloway et al. 2007).

The study used a multivariate model to calculate nitrogen associated with imports to Japan and estimated that about 2.2 Mha of foreign farmland were needed to produce annual pork and chicken imports based on the average from 2000 to 2002. Adding to this the land needed for beef and dairy product imports would end up with a total of around 3 Mha (see table 5.1; graph 5.1). In 1975 the total farmland needed to produce Japan's food was 15.8 Mha. By the year 2000, the total had grown to nearly 19 Mha. In relative terms, these totals translate, respectively, to about 1,400 and 1,500 hectares per capita, and they mean that in 1975, 65 percent of the land needed to grow Japan's food was abroad. By 2000, this share rose to 74 percent. Japan's land claim of nearly 19 Mha in 2000 was roughly equal to all of France's arable land, and in terms of its share located abroad (roughly 75 percent), it ranks first among the world's ten largest economies.

That this share is larger than the often quoted share of Japan's dependence on food imports is not surprising. The self-sufficiency ratio is calculated simply on the basis of available food energy, not on the basis of land needed to produce it. In the year 2000 it was 68 percent for dairy products, 52 percent for meat, and 40 percent for all food energy—while it was only about 25 percent in terms of arable land actually used to produce all domestic and imported food. Table 5.1 and graph 5.1 show at a glance how this came to be, from an almost complete reliance on domestic farmland in 1900 to shifting a quarter of Japan's farmland claim abroad by the mid-1930s, and then building on this base after the war and expanding the dependence on foreign arable land to nearly two-thirds by the mid-1970s and roughly three-quarters by century's end. With the currently cultivated land at less than 400 m^2/capita, it must be expected that Japan has to rely on foreign farmland in order to secure its rich and well-balanced diet. Judging the magnitude of that foreign claim—farmland amounting to about 1,100 m²/capita—is a matter of perspective.

Japan's claim is enormous when compared to China's demand, but a still very modest one when compared to the American mean. When the area needed for China's food supply is adjusted for the domestic production of nonfood crops and for the trade in plant and animal foodstuffs (China has been a major importer of soybeans, a major exporter of corn), its per capita land claim came only to about 1,100 m² in the year 2000, with only about 12 percent located abroad. When the same adjustments are done for the United States in 2000, the average claim—despite the country's enormous food exports that needed about 30 Mha, or 17 percent of all farmland—still came to 5,000 m²/capita. The average Japanese thus claims foreign farmland nearly equal to China's total per capita farmland needs, but remains a frugal food consumer when compared to the excessive food consumption and waste in the United States.

Water

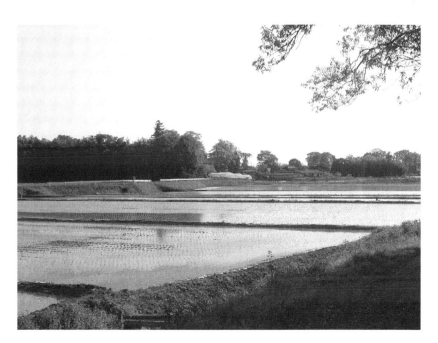

Figure 5.2
Young rice growing in a flooded field. (K. Kobayashi)

Water Needs

Photosynthesis involves an inherently lopsided exchange of CO_2 (a trace atmospheric gas whose current concentration is about 0.039 percent) and H_2O, the dominant constituent (more than 90 percent) of fresh leaves: the difference between the concentration of water vapor inside the leaves and in the ambient air is two orders of magnitude greater than the difference between external and internal levels of CO_2. That is why cultivated plants following the C_3 metabolic pathway (including the two principal food grains, wheat and rice, as well as all leguminous crops, tubers, and vegetables) need at least 900 to 1,200 moles, and some up to 4,000 moles of H_2O, to fix a single mole of CO_2, while the C_4 plants (most notably corn, sorghum, and sugarcane, whose metabolic pathway is less wasteful) require "only" 400 to 500 moles H_2O to a single mole of CO_2 fixed (Smil 2008).

Wheat plants thus need about 1,300 liters (1.3 tonnes) of water in order to produce 1 kg of grain, typical requirements for rice are about 2.3 tonnes per kg, some beans require more than 4 tonnes per kg, and lentils require around 6 tonnes per kg, (Chapagain and Hoekstra 2004). In contrast, only a very small part of the water used by photosynthesis is actually incorporated into plant tissues: grains are harvested only once their moisture drops below 20 to 25 percent and are stored and marketed with moisture levels between 10 and 15 percent. One tonne of wheat that needed 1,300 tonnes of water to produce will thus contain only about 110 kg of water. Most of the world's crops are rainfed, but water is required for regular irrigation in all arid regions (or for supplementary irrigation during dry spells in seasonally dry areas) as well as for the cultivation of paddy rice, and it can be sourced from surface waters or lifted from the ground.

Measuring the overall efficiency of irrigation is a sequential process that includes the efficiency of water storage (with reservoir losses due to evaporation and seepage), of water conveyance (quotient of water delivered to fields and the total water supplied to conduits, with most of the difference accounted for by seepage losses), and of field irrigation. This last ratio is calculated in two ways: for irrigation engineers, it is the ratio of water reaching the root zone and the total volume of water delivered to the field, while for an agronomist, it would be a quotient of evapotranspiration and delivered water. No matter how they are measured, these efficiencies were very low (often no higher than 25 percent) in traditional irrigation systems, and only the most efficient center-pivot and, even more so, drip irrigation can raise them above 70 percent.

At the same time, these calculations, done for a particular field or an irrigation system, are misleading: water lost due to seepage may be available for downstream use (as surface water or groundwater), and even water lost due to evaporation may contribute to downwind precipitation within the same watershed. As a result, overall water use efficiencies for entire watersheds are always substantially higher than for individual fields. In Japan's case, the entire concept is made even more questionable due to the multipurpose nature of the infrastructure (water reservoirs, canals, and wet fields) for crop cultivation: it provides water for other uses and acts as an important protection against floods and excessive soil erosion.

Water Resources and Flooded Fields

Water provides a notable exception to Japan's notoriously limited endowment of natural resources. The country is part of Asia's enormous monsoon regime, and hence it receives seasonally abundant precipitation: its nationwide annual mean is about 167 centimeters (compared to 108 centimeters in India, 87 in France, and 72 in the United States), and its total volume adds up to about 630 cubic kilometers a year (FAO 2011d). This produces an annual surface flow of about 420 cubic kilometers, groundwater recharge of some 27 cubic kilometers a year, and average per capita renewable water supply of nearly 3,400 cubic meters, higher than the French rate (almost 3,300 cubic meters) and well above both the Indian (less than 1,600 cubic meters) and the Chinese (2,100 cubic meters) rates. Still, droughts are possible and their frequency is higher during the years that follow the El Niño Southern Oscillation warm events than in normal years.

National agricultural water use is determined by both the prevailing climate and the crops grown. French cultivation is overwhelmingly rain fed, and only about 14 percent of the country's farmland can be irrigated, the share identical to the United States. In contrast, regional aridity in China and India combines with extensive rice cultivation to raise the share of irrigated land to, respectively, 38 percent and nearly 35 percent, while the share of Japan's paddy fields remained above half of all farm-land throughout the twentieth century. It rose from about 53 percent in 1900 (about 2.8 Mha) to peak at almost 59 percent in 1969 and then decline to about 54 percent (2.5 Mha) by 2009.

Japanese statistics also show that some 50,000 hectares of new paddies were created annually before World War II, while between 20,000 and 30,000 hectares were lost due to natural disasters, conversions to other uses, or abandonment. After the war expansion, annual rates fell rapidly since the late 1960s, and for most of the years during the last two decades of the twentieth century, they were well below 1,000 hectares; in contrast, the area of abandoned paddies remained around 20,000 hectares a year, a disparity necessarily leading to substantial cumulative losses of flooded fields. By 2000, Japan's paddies were about 23 percent below the peak reached in 1969, and this downward trend continued during the first decade of the twenty-first century.

Surface irrigation has been always dominant in Japan, and thanks to the country's mountainous terrain, all but a small part of the needed water could be drawn from streams and reservoirs by gravity. Where pumping was needed, it was traditionally accomplished by simple man-powered devices or water-powered wheels. But given the highly frag-mented nature of crop cultivation and the dominance of very small paddy fields, gravity irrigation has always depended on extensive networks of canals (whose length had greatly surpassed the overall length of the nation's highways or railways) as well as on terracing and construction of a large number of water reservoirs. Gravity irrigation could not succeed without careful management, cooperative use, and regular main-tenance of conduits (Francks 1984; Morishima 1990).

Traditionally this was often achieved through agreements needed to resolve repeated water disputes that arose during the periods of drought. During the Meiji era, water resources became a national property, and since 1896, their allocation for all uses has been administered by the state government while agricultural uses have been managed since 1949 within land improvement districts (their number now exceeds 6,000, with more than 4 million members) by participatory agreements with the beneficiaries paying the required water charges (Tanaka and Sato 2005; Okamoto 2006). By 2000, Japan's water supply system had more than 1,000 dams and 42,000 of main water channels, and it could deliver about 60 billion cubic meters per year, or two-thirds of the country's total water use (Sato 2001).

The most important change at its receiving end has been the creation of larger paddy fields. By 2000, this consolidation had created plots of at least 0.3 hectares (or 3,000 m²) on 56 percent of all paddy land—but larger plots of 1 hectare or more were still no more than 5 percent of all wet fields (Sato 2001). Due to the stagnating demand for rice and higher average rice yields, only about two-thirds of Japan's paddy fields have been planted recently with rice; the rest have been used to cultivate wheat or soybeans or left fallow. But these economic realities should not lead to a large-scale abandonment of paddies. As already noted, these fields provide important environmental services by storing heavy monsoon rainfall, reducing the risk of flooding (their aggregate storage capacity is about 5 cubic kilometers) and soil erosion, and recharging aquifers. Moreover, the need to maintain adequate levels in canals in order to deliver sufficient water to the remaining paddy fields means that even in areas where wet field cultivation has been significantly reduced, the overall water diversion from reservoirs or dams may not decrease (Yuge, Anan, and Nakano 2008).

Water for Japan's Food Production

Water needs for Japan's crop harvests are obviously dominated by the need to supply adequate water for paddy fields. Nonpaddy irrigation creates a very small part of the overall requirement: it was introduced only after World War II, and by the 1990s sprinklers were used on nearly 250,000 hectares (including cereals, vegetables, and meadows) and micro-irrigation (for vegetables, fruits, and flowers) served another 55,000 hectares—in all, just over 6 percent of all nonpaddy farmland (FAO 2011d). The two other important needs for water supply in Japan's food production are in animal husbandry and industrial-scale food processing, particularly in the meat sector, canning, and beverage production.

The total amount of water needed to grow a crop (in millimeters per day, per month, or during the entire growing season) can be estimated fairly accurately as a function of evapotranspiration and the crop factor. In turn, evapotranspiration is a function of several climatic variables, and its lowest values (just 3–4 millimeters per day with mean daily temperatures between 15°C and 25°C) are in cool, humid, and cloudy environments with minimal wind, while the rates can be twice as high in hot, arid, and windy climates. Evapotranspiration can be modeled, or it can be measured by using a standard pan evaporation method. Measurements of daytime evapotranspiration of summer and winter crops in Japan show, respectively, average rates of 3.5 and 2.5 millimeters per day, with monthly means of up to 5.7 and 6.5 millimeters per day (Attarod, Aoki, and Bayramzadeh 2009). Crop factors (crop coefficients) depend on growth stage: they are low initially, rising during the period of rapid growth, and stabilize during the midseason before declining prior to the harvest (Allen et al. 1998).

Global averages for water use by major field crops range from the lows of just above 100 cubic meters per tonne for sugar beets and silage sorghum to more than 4,000 cubic meters per tonne for lentils and millets; the rates for the three leading cereals crops—wheat, rice and corn—are, respectively, about 1,350, 2,300, and 900 cubic meters per tonne, and the highest rate apply to beverage crops, with coffee at more than 17,000, tea at nearly 25,000 and cocoa beans at more than 27,000 cubic meters per tonne (Chapagain and Hoekstra 2004). In contrast, Hoekstra and Chapagain (2007) calculated the average water use by major Japanese crops at about 1,590 cubic meters per tonne for husked rice (less than the global mean due to Japan's humid and cloudy climate) and only about 750 cubic meters per tonne for wheat but nearly 1,500 cubic meters per tonne for (often irrigated) corn. Approximate calculations of aggregate evapotransiration by Japan's food crops show the totals rising from less than 13 cubic kilometers in 1900 to about 15 cubic kilometers by 1950, peaking at about 23 cubic kilometers during the 1970s, and then falling to roughly 21 cubic kilometers by 2000.

Given the varieties of production arrangements, breeds, feeds, and typical productivities, it is inevitable that estimating water volumes needed in animal husbandry is difficult. Differences are particularly large when estimating virtual water needs, that is, water required to produce concentrate feeds (usually high-protein mixtures), high-quality forages (alfalfa, clover), and rangeland grass. Evapotranspiration of 1 cubic meter of water may produce as little as 0.5 kg of dry-matter phytomass in nonirrigated grasslands or as much as 4 to 5 kg in irrigated cultivation of forages (Molden 2007). Direct water intakes by domestic animals vary substantially by species and breed, air temperature, water content of feed, and activity. And, not surprisingly, drinking requirements nearly double in lactating cows.

Hoekstra and Chapagain (2007) published nation-specific estimates of virtual water content of animal foods produced in Japan: for the period 1997 to 2001, they were about 11,000 cubic meters per tonne of beef, 5,000 cubic meters per tonne of pork, 3,000 cubic meters per tonne of chicken, 1,900 cubic meters per tonne of eggs, and 800 cubic meters per tonne of milk. Applying these values to Japan's animal food production 2000 results in an aggregate need of about 26 cubic kilometers of water. Oki et al. (2003) used generally higher rates (in cubic meters per tonne, about 21,000 for beef, 5,900 for pork, 4,500 of chicken, 3,200 for eggs, and 560 for milk) to estimate the need of 32 cubic kilometers of virtual water for Japan's domestically produced animal foods in the year 2000. Given the inherent uncertainty of these calculations, 30 cubic kilometers may be a rough compromise value.

Simply adding this total to 21 cubic kilometers needed to grow Japan's crops would involve considerable double-counting because the virtual water that was used for the domestic production of feed and forages was already accounted for in the evapotranspiration total for crops, while virtual water used to produce imported feed will be accounted for separately in crop imports. Fortunately, starting in 1965, Japanese statistics list the totals of domestically produced and imported feed. In that year, 45 percent of all feed was imported; that share rose to about 66 percent in 1975 and 75 percent by 2000 with no significant change afterward. Consequently, adjusted virtual water demand of Japan's animal food production was about 8 cubic kilometers in 1975 and then rose to roughly 22 cubic kilometers (75 percent of 30 cubic kilometers) in 2000. Before the late 1950s, virtually all animal feed was produced domestically, but the overall output of animal foodstuffs was so small that its virtual water content (about 1 cubic kilometer in 1925 and 1.5 cubic kilometers by 1950) was smaller than the inevitable margin of error in calculating the virtual water cost of crops.

Aggregate evapotranspiration demand of Japan's domestic food production thus rose from about 13 cubic kilometers in 1900 to 17 in 1950, then it nearly doubled to 30 cubic kilometers in 1975 and rose to about 43 cubic kilometers in 2000. Inevitable storage, conveyance, and field losses mean that a substantially larger volume had to be withdrawn for irrigation. The FAO (2011d) estimated Japan's total agricultural water withdrawal at about 58 cubic kilometers during the early 1980s and at 55 cubic kilometers in 2000 (or just over 60 percent of the nation's total water consumption), with the rest roughly split between municipal and industrial uses. This demand does not impose any great burden on the country's water resources.

Total freshwater withdrawal for agriculture is less than 13 percent of the water volume that is renewable on an annual basis (FAO 2011d). For comparison, at the beginning of the twenty-first century, agricultural withdrawals accounted for 30 percent of the renewable supply in India, 15 percent in China, less than 7 percent in the United States, and a mere 2 percent in France. But due to Japan's large imports of feed and food crops, as well as substantial purchases of animal foodstuffs, it is necessary, as in the case of overall land claims, to quantify the volumes of virtual water present in the shipments of cereals, forages, legumes, oilseeds, vegetables, and fruits and in the purchases of meat and dairy products.

Virtual Water in Food and Feed Imports

The concept of virtually traded water—that is, water required for producing an imported crop or animal foodstuff as opposed to that product's actual water content—was introduced by John Anthony Allan when he tried to illustrate the magnitude of the Middle Eastern and North African water savings due to the grain imports by those arid regions (Allan 1993). The concept became widely accepted, and since the mid-1990s, the trade in virtual water has been examined in many studies at global, regional, and national scales (Hoekstra 2003; de Fraiture et al. 2004; Hoekstra and Hung 2005; Hoekstra and Chapagain 2007). Of course, the concept can be extended to virtually every traded commodity because water is needed for extracting and refining crude oil, as well as for producing steel, chemicals, and countless manufactures, but virtual water used in crop production dominates national accounts for all major economies with large substantial production.

If water is seen as the most important limiting input in intensive cropping, the concept offers an intriguing tool for global optimization of crop cultivation—but one whose use requires appropriate caveats. Global cereal trade reduces the need for irrigation water by more than 110 cubic kilometers, a major saving that is roughly equal to total annual water withdrawals in Germany, France, and Italy (de Fraiture et al. 2004). But the benefits of virtual water trade are not universal because most imports do not produce any real savings, and in other cases they can lead to higher water consumption. For example, corn, the world's leading feed crop, can be grown in the U.S. Corn Belt with just 500 cubic meters per tonne of grain, while its cultivation in Japan needs three times as much water (Hoekstra and Chapagain 2007). But this is not an excellent example of water-sparing trade because this corn (as well Japan's imports of U.S., Canadian, and Australian wheat, Brazilian soybeans, and Canadian rapeseed) is grown overwhelmingly (more than 90 percent) with rainwater rather than with irrigation water diverted from rivers, reservoirs, or aquifers.

In the absence of such crop cultivation, most of the precipitation would be evapotranspired by natural vegetation, conveyed underground, or simply evaporated from the soil surfaces. And if Japan were to import a large share of its rice from the United States, there would be no virtual water gains, while rice imported from tropical Thailand would actually evapotranspire more water than the crop grown in Japan. And while Iowa soybeans may evapotranspire twice as much water per harvested unit as Kansas wheat, that water vapor reenters the atmosphere, and if it is rapidly condensed on its way downwind, it may help to grow corn crops in Illinois or end up on farmland on another continent or in the ocean or in mountain ice. This is an obvious consequence of global water cycling, and reducing this process to a one-time task of crop-producing evapotranspiration in a given location is subtly but undeniably misleading.

Consequently, some nations that are exporting large volumes of virtual water in the form of rain-fed crops do so at no peril to their agroecosystems or their environment. Some nations importing large volumes of virtual water enjoy substantial domestic water savings (Egypt and Saudi Arabia come to mind), but others, including water-rich Japan, have made that choice for reasons other than to minimize domestic water use. Finally, the only practical way to quantify these virtual water flows is to calculate the requisite crop-specific totals of theoretically expected evapotranspiration. But if the exports come from irrigated land, it is usually impossible to estimate the actual amount of water used in the process. Doubling the evapotranspired volume, that is, assuming overall 50 percent storage, conveyance, and field efficiency, would be a good choice as the first approximation.

With these caveats in mind, here are the best available (although necessarily only approximate) quantifications of virtual water trade on the global scale and for Japanese food and feed imports. During the second half of the 1990s, the global volume of international crop-related virtual water trade annually averaged almost 700 cubic kilometers, with wheat accounting for about 30 percent of the total and virtual water in soybeans and rice amounting to about half of the volume needed to grow exported wheat. For comparison, water withdrawn for irrigation totaled about 2,600 cubic kilometers in 2000 and adding rainwater used by crops raised the grand total to at least 5,400 cubic kilometers (Hoekstra and Hung 2005). This would imply that some 13 percent of all virtual water used in crop cultivation ended up in export commodities. Not surprisingly, the United States (with its large corn, wheat, and soybean shipments) was the largest net exporter of virtual water, with about 150 cubic kilometers (or roughly 20 percent of the global total), followed by Canada, Thailand, and Argentina, all three clustering close to 50 cubic kilometers annually.

Readers of this book (aware of Japan's large cereal, soybean, oil crop, and meat imports) will not be surprised to find that Japan is by far the world's largest net importer of virtual water: its volume in the late 1990s averaged about 60 cubic kilometers a year (about 8 percent of the global total), twice the rate of second-place Netherlands (whose imports are dominated by feed for the country's cattle and pigs) and well ahead of South Korea, China, and Indonesia. A later account (Hoekstra and Chapagain 2007) put the annual global total of virtual water trade in all agricultural goods at 957 cubic kilometers for 1997 to 2001, and Japan leading with about 78 cubic kilometers. A Japanese calculation for the year 2000 (Oki et al. 2003) includes only virtual water in major cereal and leguminous grains imports (corn, wheat, rice barley, and soybeans) and in meat—the former at about 40 cubic kilometers, the latter at about 22 cubic kilometers. Because it leaves out virtual water needed to produce imports of oil crops, fruits, vegetables, and dairy products, the higher total of close to 80 cubic kilometers was a more likely volume.

Adding this total to virtual water used in domestic crop and animal food production gives a grand total of about 110 cubic kilometers in 2000, with imports accounting for 70 percent. Their share would be even higher if the total also included virtual water used in the production of seafood. The global volume of virtual water in traded seafood was estimated by Zimmer and Renault (2003) at about 200 cubic kilometers in the year 2000 (or roughly 15 percent of 1,340 cubic kilometers needed to produce all food products traded worldwide), and as Japan imported in that year about 14 percent of the globally exported fishery commodities, its share would be then roughly 28 cubic kilometers and the grand total of virtual water requirements for Japan's food supply (including about 21 cubic kilometers for the production of seafood caught or cultured by Japanese enterprises) would then rise to roughly 160 cubic kilometers, with two-thirds coming from abroad.

Nitrogen

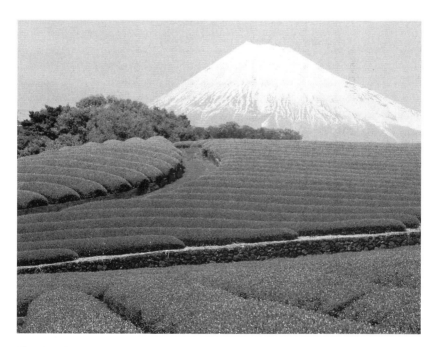

Figure 5.3
No other crop in Japan receives as much nitrogen fertilizer as tea: the highest rates used to surpass 1 tonne per hectare. This picturesque tea plantation is in Shizuoka prefecture, Japan's leading producer of *cha*. (Hiromasa Tanaka)

Nitrogen Inputs

Complexities and dynamic interdependencies of plant growth in general and crop cultivation in particular make it impossible to rank the requisite inputs of resources in any clear, meaningful order. High yields require adequate water supply; optimal amounts of phosphorus, potassium, and mineral micronutrients; as well as improved seed varieties and, if needed, applications of pesticides and herbicides. But with the exception of arid areas (where water supply is the key determinant of yields), nitrogen is almost always *primus inter pares*. No other plant macronutrient is needed in such quantities, an order of magnitude more than for phosphorus (P) and potassium (K) fertilizers, and can result in such productivity gains.

And while the biosphere is bathed in nitrogen (N_2 makes up nearly 80 percent of the atmosphere, O_2 most of the rest), nitrogenous compounds that can be absorbed by plants are comparatively scarce. This is because atmospheric N_2 is highly stable, while reactive nitrogenous compounds are highly mobile. N_2 can be split by only a few natural processes: lightning, ozonization, and, above all, specialized enzymes of *Rhizobium* bacteria that form nodules on the roots of leguminous plants. Reactive nitrogen compounds that are formed afterward through nitrogen fixation (starting with the formation of ammonia) are doubly mobile (through air and water) as ammonia is lost from the root zone by volatilization and nitrates (formed from ammonia by bacterial nitrification) are both leached into surface and ground waters and lost into the atmosphere through denitrification.

Traditional agricultures had two options to supply nitrogen: recycling organic matter (crop residues and animal and human wastes) or cultivating leguminous crops whose roots have symbiotic nitrogen-fixing bacteria. Recycling could sustain high yields, but because of low nitrogen concentrations of the recycled materials and high volatilization and leaching losses, it has been necessary to apply massive amounts of organic wastes, often more than 10 tonnes per hectare. Cultivation of leguminous cover crops (green manures that were plowed under) supplied large amounts of nitrogen (hundreds of kg per hectare) to food crops that followed them—but obviously it precluded (for periods of several months) cultivation of another food crop.

These constraints were removed only by the introduction of large-scale industrial fixation of nitrogen by the Haber-Bosch process in 1913 and the adoption of intensive cultivation based on applications of high rates of nitrogen fertilizer after World War II (Smil 2001). Traditional Japanese farming was a paragon of intensive organic recycling, resulting in rice yields that were exceptionally high for the preindustrial period. Modern Japanese farming has been highly dependent on intensive application of synthetic nitrogen fertilizers in order to maintain very high yields from a limited amount of arable land. And as in the case of land and water, where imported foodstuffs make a greater claim on the two resources than in the case of domestic cultivation, Japanese food imports have contained increasing quantities of virtual nitrogen.

Nitrogen in Japanese Agriculture

High productivity of the traditional Japanese farming rested on assiduous recycling of all possible organic wastes, including human feces and urine. In the country's largest city, the practice was formally organized during the early Edo period (Tanaka 1998; Ministry of Environment 2008). In 1649, the capital's rulers ordered the dismantling of all toilets that were directly discharging waste into rivers and moats and ordered payment for night soil removal. By 1662 disposal companies were taking away virtually all of the generated waste to suburban fields. Steps were taken to set up night soil reservoirs near fields in order to ferment the wastes and convert them to pathogen-free fertilizer.

Nearly 250 years later, Japan's Western residents during the Meiji era would describe the practice as basically unchanged. In 1890 Chamberlain wrote that among many recycled wastes used as fertilizer, "the commonest is night soil, whose daily conveyance all about the country causes no distress to native noses" (Chamberlain 1890, 20). This recycling remained a major source of nitrogen until after World War II when widespread availability of synthetic high-nitrogen fertilizers (urea's nitrogen content is two orders of magnitude that of nightsoil or compost) made it much easier to supply the needed nutrient with applications of just tens or hundreds of kg of fertilizer per hectare rather than fermenting, transporting and applying more than 10 tonnes per hectare and, not uncommonly even more than 30 tonnes per hectare, of organic wastes.

But in overall mass terms, the largest supply of nitrogen came from composts containing various shares of animal manures, crop residues (mostly rice straw), and other organic wastes. Plants were also collected in nearby mountains and grasslands and applied to paddy soils to supply nutrients, a practice that often resulted in degraded plant cover and reduced soil organic matter and, hence, led to greater flood risks. The third indispensable source of nitrogen came from planting green manures—most commonly, the Chinese milk vetch *(Astragalus sinicus)*, soybeans, broad beans, and alfalfa—that were plowed in after a few months of cultivation in order to provide nitrogen for the subsequent food crop. Many crop residues, above all, rice straw, were also plowed in after the harvest, but a great deal of straw was not recycled (directly or indirectly in animal feed and bedding) because it was used for thatching and making sandals, hats, coats, *tatami*, rope, and bales or because it was used for household fuel or burned in the field.

Nearly all of these organic materials have very low nitrogen content, ranging most commonly between 0.5 and 0.6 percent for night soil as well as for stable manures and green manures. The only materials with considerably higher share of nitrogen were oilseed cakes (soybean cakes have up to 6.5 percent nitrogen) and, in coastal regions, fertilizer made from sardines and herrings (more than 9 percent nitrogen). Domestic production of oilseed cakes could never cover a potentially huge domestic demand for these relatively concentrated sources of organic nitrogen, and imports of soybean cakes for fertilizer began in 1895, immediately after the end of the Sino-Japanese War, and within a decade they were above 150,000 tonnes per year (Deschamp 1911). However, a large part of this organic nitrogen was used in sericulture (for mulberry cultivation) and in production of such cash crops as cotton and indigo, rather than in food production.

There are some rough estimates for total applications of major organic fertilizers during the pre–World War II period and they can be used, together with realistic assumptions about their average nitrogen content (using conservative means of 0.5 percent nitrogen for night soil and green manures and 0.3 percent for composts), to calculate the overall inputs of recycled nitrogen in Japan's crop cultivation during the early decades of the twentieth century. In 1900 all organic fertilizers supplied at least 170,000 tonnes of nitrogen. By 1925 the total applications of composts reached about 22 Mt and those of night soil about 16 Mt while green manures added about 6 Mt and other materials a further 8 Mt, for a total of roughly 250,000 tonnes of nitrogen. A decade later, the total amount of nitrogen rose, mostly due to a further expansion of composting, to about 300,000 tonnes.

To this must be added nitrogen fixed by *Rhizobium* bacteria symbiotic with leguminous food crops (mainly soybeans and various beans) as well as nitrogen added to soils by free living fixers (mostly cyanobacteria) in both paddy and dry fields. Free-living fixers may add annually as little nitrogen as 5 kg per hectare but up to 40 kg per hectare in paddy fields, most beans do not add more than 25 kg per hectare, but a soybean crop can leave behind as much as 60 to 100 kg per hectare (Smil 2001). Applying conservative nitrogen fixation averages to the areas planted to paddy rice, soybeans, other legumes and other crops results in annual fixation of nitrogen of at least 125,000 tonnes in 1900, 130,000 in 1925, and 140,000 in 1950. The final two inputs of nitrogen before the advent of inorganic fertilizers were in precipitation and irrigation water. At the beginning of the twentieth century, the first input of nitrogen was negligible, while the second input contributed at least 15,000 tonnes in 1900 and as much as 30,000 by 1950.

Japan's use of commercial fertilizers began with the imports of relatively small quantities of guano, Chilean nitrates, and ammonium sulfate (as well as phosphates) during the late nineteenth century, and by 1910 the value of fertilizer imports accounted for about a tenth of all foreign purchases. The first two imports reached their peaks by 1920 with nearly 16,000 tonnes of guano and more than 122,000 tonnes of nitrate, but imports of ammonium sulfate continued to grow, reaching more than 200,000 tonnes per year by the 1930s. In 1908 Shitagau Noguchi and Joichi Fujiyama set up Nippon Chisso Hiryō (Japan Fertilizer Company), which half a century later became infamous as the source of mercury in Minamata poisoning (its cause was first recognized in November 1956), and in 1909 it began to use the German process for synthesizing calcium cyanamide, $CaCN_2$ (Japan Fertilizer and Ammonia Producers Association 2010).

The first small plant using the Haber-Bosch ammonia process, commercialized in Germany by 1913, began to produce ammonium sulfate in 1923 and the first domestic version of the synthesis succeeded by 1931. By 1920 cyanamide output was above 100,000 tonnes a year, and the production of ammonium sulfate had surpassed 600,000 tonnes a year by 1935 (IIA 1937). Using the standard conversion ratios of 21

Table 5.2
Nitrogen in Japanese food supply, 1900–2000

| Year | Fertilizers | | | Crop residues | Precipitation | Biofixation | Irrigation | Total domestic nitrogen input |
	Organic	Inorganic	Total					
1900	0.17	0.01	0.18	0.05	0.02	0.12	0.01	0.3861
1925	0.25	0.10	0.35	0.06	0.03	0.13	0.02	0.5985
1950	0.20	0.40	0.60	0.07	0.03	0.15	0.03	0.88
1975	0.50	0.65	1.15	0.15	0.04	0.15	0.05	1.54
2000	0.35	0.49	0.84	0.15	0.03	0.13	0.03	1.18

Synthetic nitrogen fertilizers used to produce domestic and imported food, 1900–2000

| Year | Domestic applications | Virtual nitrogen in imported | | Total nitrogen | Share of foreign contributions (percent) |
		Crops	Animal foods		
1900	0.05	—	—	0.05	0
1925	0.10	0.05	—	0.15	33
1950	0.37	0.10	—	0.47	21
1975	0.65	0.65	0.20	1.50	56
2000	0.49	1.00	0.45	1.94	75

Note: All values, except for the last column, are in Mt of nitrogen.

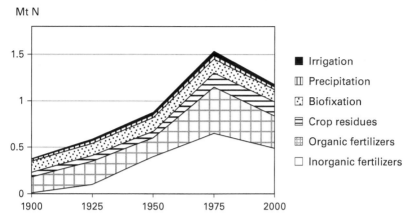

Mt N

Irrigation
Precipitation
Biofixation
Crop residues
Organic fertilizers
Inorganic fertilizers

Graph 5.2
Total nitrogen inputs in Japan's agriculture for 1900–2000.

percent of nitrogen for ammonium sulfate, 20 percent in calcium cyanamide, and 16 percent for Chilean nitrate (Smil 2001) and assuming 5
percent N in imported guano, results in the total consumption of about
10,000 tonnes of nitrogen in commercial fertilizers in 1900 and 100,000
tonnes in 1925 (table 5.2; graph 5.2). By 1940 the total rose to over
250,000 tonnes.

By 1950 the use of all kinds of synthetic nitrogenous fertilizers reached
nearly 370,000 tonnes of nitrogen, and the subsequent expansion of rice
harvests drove the rapid increase in nitrogen applications to a peak of
775,900 tonnes in 1967. After a slight dip came another peak in 1979
(777,000 tonnes), but by 1985, nitrogen fertilizer applications were
down to 680,000 tonnes and then a combination of declining rice harvests and improved uptake efficiencies lowered the annual rate to less
than 500,000 tonnes by the year 2000 (figure 5.3; graph 5.2). There was
a concurrent decline in the provision of organic nitrogen due to a combination of fewer domestic animals, a falling share of recycled manure,
a smaller cropland area in general, and reduced planting of legumes in
particular.

We have a representative survey of soil nitrogen status in Japan's
agricultural soils thanks to an analysis of nearly 150 plow-layer samples
collected from both paddy and dry fields in every part of the country
(Sano, Yanai, and Kosaki 2004). Results of this survey were analyzed
according to the nutrient's form and availability, and they showed that

nitrogen content averaging 2.5 grams of nitrogen per kilogram, with the available fraction (extractable inorganic and mineralizable organic nitrogen) being less than 8 percent of total stores and the stable fraction (fixed NH_4-N and the element embedded in long-lived organic compounds) forming the rest. The available nitrogen fraction prorated to about 295 kg of nitrogen per hectare , comparable to actual total annual nitrogen inputs in organic recycling, biofixation, and commercial fertilizers. This means that Japan's agricultural soils are, on average, fairly rich in available nitrogen.

Nitrogen for Domestic and Imported Food

Any reasonably complete account of nitrogen flows in a national agroecosystem can be nothing more than a very rough approximation of complex realities. Only two fluxes of the entire set (application of synthetic fertilizers and the nutrient's removal in harvested crops and their residues) are known with a high degree of certainty. All other flows must be estimated by using what appear to be best, and often compounded, assumptions whose reliability ranges from acceptable (shares of recycled animal manures and crop residues, nitrogen in precipitation) to unsatisfactory (actual rates of biofixation by symbiotic and free-living bacteria, typical rates of denitrification).

Rice has always received most of the applied nitrogen, and during the 1970s and the 1980s, there were many studies of the best fertilization practices and efficiency of nitrogen uptake in paddy fields (International Rice Research Institute 1979, 1987; de Datta and Patrick 1983). Toriyama's (2002) experiments established that the Japanese rice yielding of 5 tonnes per hectare (this is in terms of brown, husked, rice and is an equivalent of about 6 tonnes per hectare of paddy rice) needs 73 kg N/ha for single-cropped paddy and 112 kg N/ha for double-cropped fields. During the last decade of the twentieth century, most of this demand was supplied by synthetic fertilizers followed by organic recycling, bacterial nitrogen fixation with nitrogen dissolved in irrigation water, and precipitation being the least important contributions.

However, rice has not been the crop that has been receiving the highest applications per area of nitrogen. Intensive multicropping of such common vegetables as cabbages or daikon may require 100 to 150 kg of nitrogen per hectare for every crop and hence the annual total may surpass 300 or even 500 kg , and leafy vegetables cultivated under plastic covers or in greenhouses receive 300–600 kg N and as much as 500 kg of N/ha can be used for eggplants, melons, tomatoes, and onions (Kumazawa 2002; Mishima 2001), and yet even these extraordinarily high rates are far below the applications used in intensive cultivation of tea.

The quality (and hence the price) of Japan's green tea is related to its high theanin (an amino acid) content, and that is why, since the mid-1970s, its cultivation has been practiced with excess applications of fertilizer (Yokota, Morita, and Ghanati 2005). Tea plantations in Shizuoka prefecture, Japan's leading tea-growing area, received about 100 kg of nitrogen per hectare at the beginning of the twentieth century (virtually all of it in organic wastes), up to 400 kg by the mid-1960s, 800 kg/ha two decades later and more than 1,000 kg/ha (and in some cases even 2,500 kg/ha) of nitrogen per hectare during the early 1990s; only then was the practice reformed, and the rates fell to around 600 kg after 2000 (Oh et al. 2006; Hirono, Watanabe, and Nonaka 2009). Even lower applications (about 400 kg of nitrogen per hectare) are possible when using calcium cyanamide, and they also prevent further soil acidification (some tea fields had soils with pH below 3). Wheat and sweet potatoes are two other major crops that have been receiving high fertilizer applications (often in excess of 100 kg of nitrogen per hectare).

The best Japanese quantifications of agricultural nitrogen flows during the last twenty years of the twentieth century (Mishima, Matsumoto, and Oda 1999; Mishima 2001) were based on a wide range of relevant statistical data, and they are obviously less inaccurate than are the merely suggestive reconstructions that trace some basic trends for the years 1900, 1925, and 1950 (all of these estimates are summarized in table 5.2). In 1900 Japan's agroecosystem received about 400,000 tonnes of nitrogen; about 55 percent of this total were recycled organic wastes, about 30 percent came from biofixation and less than 3 percent from inorganic fertilizers. By 1925 the total rose to about 600,000 tonnes N, with recycling contributing about half, biofixation about one-fifth, and inorganic fertilizers at least 15 percent. By 1950 the share of synthetic fertilizers reached 45 percent, and recycling contributed less than a third of the overall input of some 880,000 tonnes. Mishima's (2001) calculations show the total input of nearly 1.3 Mt N by 1980 (with 45 percent from synthetic fertilizers) and at least 1.1 Mt for the late 1990s (with about 40 percent supplied by inorganic compounds).

These realities have a number of interesting and important implications. Because of the post-1950 surge in fertilizer inputs, Japan had joined a small group of countries whose average applications of inorganic nitrogen compounds had surpassed 100 kg of N/ha. The Netherlands had reached that level before World War II, and by 1950 the Dutch mean was nearly 160 kg; Japan surpassed the 100 kilogram mark in 1954; Egypt joined the group by 1969 and China by 1979 (Smil 2001). Many field studies have shown that the overall nitrogen uptake efficiency is generally higher for organic sources of nitrogen (as long as they are appropriately incorporated into soil) than for inorganic compounds and that the uptake of synthetic fertilizers declines with higher rates of application.

Both of these conclusions are confirmed by the approximate nitrogen flow data for 1900 to 2000. Early in the twentieth century, when most nitrogen came from organic sources, the overall uptakes were on the order of 50 to 60 percent compared to the rates of no better than 40 to 45 percent between the 1950s and the 1970s, while the reduced applications of synthetic fertilizers after 1980 were accompanied by a continuing rise in yields and hence by more efficient nitrogen utilization. This change is best seen with rice fertilization. Japan's actual fertilizer applications to paddy rice were rising fairly linearly, from about 50 kg in 1940 to 100 kg of nitrogen per hectare in 1960 and then they peaked around 110 kg in mid-1980s; afterward, as the uptake efficiency improved, they fell to about 85 kg in 1995 and even to less than 70 kg of nitrogen per hectare in 2003 (Mishima, Taniguchi, and Komada 2006). This decline in fertilizer application to rice paddies could be partly due to the transition of rice from the dominant staple to a luxury foodstuff; better palatability of cooked rice and the quest for a higher market price have been other considerations that led to reduced application of nitrogen fertilizer in Japan's paddies.

Given Japan's high dependence on food imports, it is necessary, as was done in the case of farmland and water needed for crop cultivation, to add virtual nitrogen—that is, the nutrient used in producing the imported foodstuffs but not physically contained in the shipped products (that would be the embedded nitrogen)—to Japan's overall nutrient flow. Again, this is a relatively straightforward task in the case of imported crops and plant foods: their weights are simply multiplied by appropriate rates of average nitrogen applications in the exporting countries. In contrast, calculating how much nitrogen had to be used to grow feed for imported meat and dairy products is a much more difficult challenge whose best outcomes are approximations with an inevitably significant margin of possible errors.

One way to reduce the overall uncertainty is to limit the quantification of virtual nitrogen to applications of synthetic fertilizers because the information on their recommended use in crop and plant food exporting countries is readily available in relevant national and international (mainly FAO) agronomic literature. Virtual inorganic nitrogen present in Japan's limited imports of wheat, rice, and sugar was negligible in 1900 (less than 5,000 tonnes), it reached no more than 50,000 tonnes in 1925, and 100,000 tonnes by 1950. Subsequent expansion of imports brought the total to about 650,000 tonnes by 1975 and approximately 1 Mt in 2000. To this must be added much less accurate estimates of nitrogen needed to produce imported animal foods.

An already noted study of international meat trade (Galloway et al. 2007) found that during the years 2000 to 2002, virtual nitrogen in the Japanese imports of pork and chicken amounted to about 220,000 tonnes, with half of it used in the production of the U.S. exports. Pork and chicken accounted for roughly half of all Japanese imports of animal protein, and hence a rough estimate of all virtual nitrogen in meat and dairy imports would be on the order of 440,000 tonnes. This simple multiplication ignores two opposing realities: a relatively high protein conversion efficiency in milk production (more than 30 percent of all digested nitrogen ends up in milk) and a low conversion efficiency in producing beef (less than 10 percent of digested nitrogen ends up in meat). Nevertheless, a disaggregated accounting of these differences (including the weighted average of the two conversions) results in a very similar overall figure of about 460,000 tonnes of nitrogen for the year 2000. Annual means for the period 1975 to 1980 were no more than 200,000 tonnes, and for the decades before 1970, they were negligible (much smaller than unavoidable error margins of these calculations).

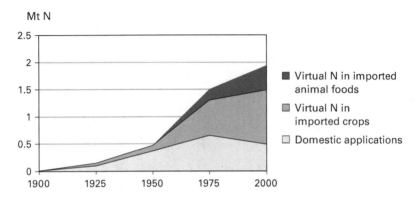

Graph 5.3
Synthetic nitrogen fertilizers used to produce domestic and imported foods, 1900–2000.

Now it is possible to present the final account of Japan's demand for commercial fertilizer nitrogen (leaving out all organic recycling and biofixation) during the twentieth century (graph 5.3). Domestic use of fertilizers rose from no more than 10,000 tonnes of nitrogen in 1900 (all imported) to about 100,000 tonnes in 1925 when virtual nitrogen in imported crops amounted to about 50,000 tonnes, or a third of the total. By 1950 domestic fertilizer use rose to 370,000 tonnes of nitrogen and virtual nitrogen reached 100,000 tonnes, or roughly a fifth of the total input. By 1975 domestic applications of nitrogenous fertilizers had nearly doubled to 650,000 tonnes of nitrogen but virtual nitrogen increased much faster—to 600,000 tonnes in imported crops and about 200,000 tonnes in imported animal foodstuffs—and it accounted for roughly 55 percent of the total supply.

Finally, by the century's end, domestic fertilizer use fell back to less than 490,000 tonnes of nitrogen, but virtual nitrogen reached 1 Mt in crops and nearly half a milliontonnes in animal foods, providing 75 percent of all the total nutrient flow consumed by Japan's food supply (table 5.2). Obviously, these changing trends had important environmental consequences because most of the nitrogen involved in crop and animal food production does not end up embedded in harvested plant organs (seeds, tubers, stalks, fruits) but escapes into the surrounding environment (be it into the atmosphere or into water), where its reactive compounds create a variety of problems.

Reactive Nitrogen in the Environment

Crop fertilization has inevitable environmental consequences because nitrogenous compounds are subject to several physical and chemical transformations that move them from soils to the atmosphere and to ground, stream, lake, and ocean waters. The two principal ways in which reactive nitrogen compounds enter the atmosphere are volatilization and denitrification. Volatilization from soils, plants, manures, and ammoniacal fertilizers adds NH_3 to the atmosphere: the gas is transported downwind and redeposited on land in rain or in dry form. Ammonia volatilization from paddy fields is primarily a function of overall urea applications and soil pH, and the losses may be only a fraction of a percent of the applied nutrient in the Japanese environment (Hayashi, Nishimura, and Yagi 2006).

Denitrification is promoted by high concentrations of nitrate, soil organic matter, moisture, and temperature and by low oxygen levels because it does not always proceed all the way to the inert N_2 and it produces significant amounts of NO and N_2O. NO takes place in various tropospheric reactions, while N_2O is unreactive in the troposphere but its stratospheric conversion to NO sets off a catalytic destruction cycle of O_3. Moreover, N_2O is also a greenhouse gas considerably more potent (two orders of magnitude) than CO_2. The best estimates are that by 2009, N_2O was responsible for just over 6 percent of the overall anthropogenic radiative forcing (World Meteorological Organization 2010).

Ammonia is not highly water soluble, and that is why most of the waterborne losses of applied fertilizers (be they organic wastes or synthetic compounds) are leached highly soluble nitrates; soil erosion can be also a major reason for waterborne nitrogen losses. Concentration of waterborne nitrates usually shows the highest correlation with the application of nitrogenous fertilizers. Nitrogen is usually the limiting macronutrient in aquatic ecosystems, and its addition causes eutrophication, enhanced growth of algae or phytoplankton whose subsequent decomposition removes oxygen from water and kills many aquatic species, above all the benthic fauna. Worst of all, this process creates offshore dead zones, large areas of hypoxic water in shallow coastal seas. Algal blooms also interfere with water filtration and can produce harmful toxins.

Given the intensity of nitrogen applications in Japan's crop cultivation (as well as the increasing numbers of relatively large-scale animal feeding operations producing large volumes of organic wastes), it is not surprising that a great deal of attention has been paid to nitrogen flows associated with the country's food production and the resulting nitrogen balances (Minami 2005; Mishima, Taniguchi, and Komada 2006; Mishima, Endo, and Kohyama 2009; He et al. 2009) and to nitrogen fertilization and nitrate pollution in particular (Kumazawa 2002; Minami 2005; Fukushima 2007).

Only a few Japanese crops have nitrogen balances—differences between all fertilizer applications, biofixation, atmospheric deposition and nitrogen in seeds and irrigation water on one hand and nitrogen removed in harvested crops and grass and fodder production—lower than 100 kg of nitrogen per hectare a, with the highest values in excess of not only 200 kg a (carrots, cabbages, taro, burdock) but even more than 500 kg of nitrogen per hectarea for tea (Kumazawa 2002). And during the last two decades of the twentieth century, even the country's nationwide average was well above that mark. International comparison shows Japan with a balance of nearly 145 kg of nitrogen per hectare during the late 1980s and about 135 kg during the years 1995 to 1997, the fourth highest rate in the Organization for Economic Cooperation and Development (2001) behind the Netherlands (about 260 kg of nitrogen per hectare), South Korea, and Belgium. Although there can be no single uniform threshold for undesirable environmental impacts, it appears that annual surpluses in excess of 30 to 70 kg of nitrogen per hectare may have negative effect on water quality.

In order to appreciate the intensity and extent of Japan's nitrate pollution, it is necessary to keep in mind the importance of groundwater and a few key contamination rates. At the beginning of the twenty-first century about 22 percent of Japan's water consumption for daily life came from ground sources, with the rate exceeding 40 percent in several regions including inland Kanto, southern Kyūshū, and the island of Shikoku (Fukushima 2007). Uncontaminated waters contain less than 0.1 mg NO_3-N/L, clean streams carry less than 1 milligram of nitrogen per liter (mg N/L), concentrations in streams contaminated by agricultural runoff commonly range from a few to more than 10 mg N/L, drinking water should have less than 10 mg N/L, and highly contaminated groundwater can have concentrations in excess of 20 mg N/L. During the early 1960s, rivers draining not only a large part of Hokkaidō but also most of the other three large islands had nitrate concentration below 1 mg N/L; in contrast, by 1998, twelve prefectural averages had river nitrate levels above 2 mg N/L (Shindo et al. 2009).

By 1990 nitrate concentrations in the groundwater used for irrigation averaged just over 10 mg N/L for dry fields and nearly 6 mg N/L for all irrigated cropland, while the highest levels in shallow wells near tea plantations or in groundwater in some upland fields and greenhouse areas were above 20 or even 30 mg N/L (Kumazawa 2002; Hirono, Watanabe and Nonaka 2009). A survey done between 2000 and 2005 found excess nitrate in nearly 6 percent of all wells, with regional averages ranging between 0 and 25 percent (Mishima, Endo, and Kohyama 2009)—and fertilization was by far the most important identifiable cause of this contamination, followed by the dumping of untreated livestock wastes (Fukushima 2007). Livestock excreta peaked in 1990 and were nearly 20 percent lower by the year 2005, with a declining share of these wastes properly recycled, with total manure applications falling from about 180,000 tonnes of nitrogen in 1990 to less than 110,000 tonnes by 2005 (Mishima, Endo, and Kohyama 2008).

The problem of excessive nitrate losses does not have any easy solutions: reducing the inputs is obviously the best approach, followed by optimized agronomic practices. Such technical fixes as fertilizers with added nitrification inhibitors, compounds with low water solubility and delayed nitrogen release, and fertilizers coated with low-permeability films (sulfur-coated urea) work fairly well but are too expensive and have found limited markets in growing garden and greenhouse vegetables, fruits, and flowers (Wakimoto 2004; Minami 2005). And Japan's excessive nitrogen loading would be much worse if it were not for the country's large food and feed imports.

Three times as much nitrogen fertilizer was used to grow Japan's cereal, oilseed, vegetable, fruit, and other plant food imports than it was applied to domestic crops, and according to calculations by Galloway et al. (2007) about 220,000 tonnes of nitrogen were left abroad due to Japan's meat imports, again about three times the amount of the nutrient that was released into Japan's environment in disposed livestock excreta that were not recycled as manure to fields. Not surprisingly, Murano et al. (1995) found that overall ammonia emissions were relatively small compared to most European countries with their higher density of cattle.

Food from the Sea

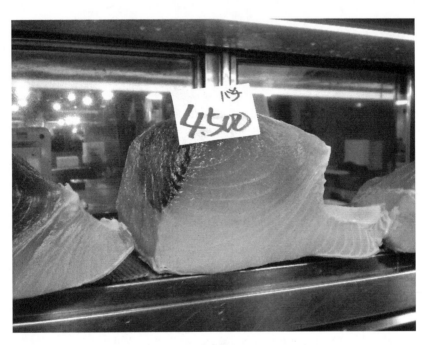

Figure 5.4
A chunk of tuna in a display case in Tsukiji, the world's largest fish market, in Tokyo. (V. Smil)

Japan led the world in total seafood capture and production for all but the last decade of the twentieth century. In terms of total landings (including aquatic plants, all marine invertebrates, and mammals), it lost this primacy to China's expanding fisheries and mariculture in 1991, and when the comparison is limited to marine fish catches, China surpassed Japan in 1994 (FAO 2011e). Subsequently, Japan's total landings of fish, crustaceans, and mollusks was surpassed by Peru (in 1999), the United States (in 2001), and Indonesia and Chile (in 2004), demoting the country to sixth place worldwide by 2005. But even then Japan remained the world's largest per capita consumer of seafood because the declining domestic landings were largely made up by rising imports.

These imports do not involve just a few most commonly consumed species but have become so broadly based that one of the greatest diversities of aquatic zoomass (unfortunately, all of it dead) can be found inside the sheds at Tsukiji, Tokyo's famous central fish market (Bestor 2004). Japan now claims significant shares of virtually every major fishery commodity, ranging from the largest carnivorous fish (all tuna species) to the smallest herbivorous species (sardines and smelt), and including marine invertebrates (squid, mussels), and (with Denmark, Iceland, and Norway as its only Western allies in that quest) the country still favors the killing of whales. These realities make it inevitable that Japan's seafood consumption figures prominently in all appraisals of the overall sustainability of global fisheries and in debates about acute overfishing of particular species, excessive exploitation of entire fishing zones, or the status and recovery of sea mammals.

They also make it difficult to confine these concerns strictly to dispassionate appraisals, conclusions, and recommendations. Japanese participants in these debates feel that the Western critics do not sufficiently acknowledge Japan's traditional, and exceptional, dependence on wild ocean species and that they display cultural insensitivity and a double standard when they see nothing wrong with the annual slaughter of tens of millions of large domesticated mammals (the United States slaughters about 35 million head of cattle and more than 110 million pigs annually) and billions of birds (recently just over 9 billion chicken in the United States) but insisting on a complete ban on hunting all whales (the species that are not listed as endangered).

Each of these claims is open to argument. On one hand, it is obvious that killing endangered stocks of wild mammals is not the same as slaughtering domesticated species whose numbers can be multiplied at will. But on the other hand, Western countries have an extraordinarily poor record in preventing excessive harvests of aquatic species under their jurisdiction and management. Nevertheless, the basic facts are undeniable: for nearly a century, Japan has had a major role in the advancing depletion of fish stocks, first in certain areas of the Pacific Ocean and after World War II worldwide. Japan's high fish consumption has had an impact on the largest carnivorous species in general and on the bluefin, the most overfished species of tuna, in particular.

The aggregate impact of Japanese whaling is a different matter. Continuation of limited Japanese whaling, ostensibly for research reasons, has been attracting a great deal of foreign criticism, but in cumulative historic terms, the whaling fleets of other nations had killed far more of the world's largest mammals. Japan's first modern whaling ship was purchased only in 1899, and its long-distance Antarctic whale hunts began only during the late 1930s. In contrast, European whalers had been active for centuries, U.S. ships were hunting whales around the world since the late eighteenth century, and Norwegians, the British, and Russian were generally more active in the post-1945 Antarctic whaling than the Japanese were (Starbuck 1989; Whaling Library 2010).

That is why Japan's cumulative whale kill remains far below the aggregate European or U.S. numbers. Yet at the same time, no other country has killed as many whales (more than 10,000 until 2007, or 40 percent of the total, with Norway in the second place) since the International Whaling Commission's moratorium on commercial hunting went into effect in 1986–1987. An annual whale hunt, carried out in the Antarctic waters as well as in North Pacific, is done ostensibly for research. But as Clapham et al. (2007) pointed out, by spring 2006 Japanese whalers had already killed nearly five times as many animals for research than have all other nations combined since 1952—and nonlethal studies of the foraging behavior of whales have produced, with far fewer resources, more definitive information (Corkeron 2009).

And while Japan's total seafood landings as well as overall consumption have declined after reaching their respective peaks (in 1984 at 11.5 Mt and in 1988 with 13.5 Mt), a combination of rising Japanese fish imports and a newly found worldwide popularity of sushi and *sashimi* (part of a broader shift toward increased consumption of seafood driven by health concerns and rising incomes) have more than made up for this decrease. But this quintessentially Japanese dietary mainstay, no matter how much it is nutritionally desirable and individually preferable, cannot be a global model. If even only a quarter of the world's population tried to emulate Japan's high per capita seafood consumption, global fish stocks would become depleted even faster than it is envisaged by today's depressing scenarios.

Japanese Catches

During the early Meiji decades, Japan continued its traditional practice of fishing restricted to coastal waters of the Sea of Japan and the Pacific Ocean. The first opportunity for territorial expansion of Japanese catches came with the occupation of Taiwan and Liaodong peninsula as a result of the Sino-Japanese War of 1894–1895, soon followed by gains during the Russo-Japanese War (1904–1905). After World War I Japan was awarded the control of the former German Pacific colonies north of the equator, the Marshall Islands, the Marianas, and the Palau Islands, where it established bases for tuna fishing (Gillett 2007). In addition, the progressing motorization of fishing vessels (first with gasoline engines, eventually with diesels) began to extend the operating ranges of Japan's fishing fleets and by the late 1930s their activities ranged from the South China Sea to the Bering Sea and encompassed a substantial part of the Pacific Ocean southeast of the Japanese islands.

Japan's historical statistics list total marine catches going all the way back to 1894, although with questionable accuracy, down to a single tonne: 1,570,562 tonnes in 1900, 2,901,566 tonnes in 1925, 3,526,016 tonnes in 1940, and the prewar record landings amounting to about 4,327,981 tonnes in 1936. During the last prewar years, the country's fisheries employed about 1.5 million people and 45 percent of the world's fishing boats were Japanese (Espenshade 1949). For comparison, during the 1930s, the United States was the second most important fishing nation and its prewar landings also peaked in 1936 at about 2.2 Mt, or only about half of Japan's catch (U.S. Bureau of the Census 1975).

Wartime destruction of vessels and ports reduced the Japanese catch to 1.8 Mt in 1945 and the Supreme Commander of occupation forces imposed restrictions on the operation of Japanese fishing vessels, limiting the country's fishing fleet to only about 40 percent of the area in the Pacific that it accessed before the war. Easing of these restrictions in 1946 and again in 1949 led to a rapid recovery of fish catches, promoted by the occupation authorities in order to improve the supply of much-needed protein: total landings were up to 2.5 Mt by 1948 and 3.37 Mt in 1950. All restrictions were removed with the signing of the 1952 peace treaty, and Japan was free to embark on a worldwide expansion of fishing. The timing could not have been better for at least four reasons.

First, Japan's rapidly expanding metallurgical and shipbuilding industries could supply large numbers of modern fishing vessels (prewar fishing vessel capacity was surpassed already in 1949). Second, the 1950s and the 1960s were the two decades of very cheap crude oil, and the vessels, equipped with efficient marine diesel engines, could be operated inexpensively even on distant journeys to rich fishing grounds in the other hemisphere. Third, there were no labor force shortages: Japan's population kept expanding, and fishing fleets could be manned with young local crews that did not demand high wages. Fourth, and perhaps most important, the national sovereignty of many coastal nations extended only up to 3 nautical miles from the shore, and rest of the ocean was open for an essentially uncontrolled exploitation. Japanese fishers took advantage of this by exploiting many distant and rich fishing grounds on major continental shelves and in upwelling areas.

By 1960, when the total annual landings were 5.8 Mt, Japan's fishing activities extended to the Pacific waters surrounding Australia (particularly to the southern region of the eastern Indian Ocean), the central Atlantic (between the Caribbean and Africa, with the heaviest concentration in the upwelling region along the African coast between Senegal and Gibraltar), and the Pacific into the Bering Sea in the north and the Southern Ocean east of New Zealand (Swartz 2000). Rising incomes kept pushing up the domestic demand for seafood, and a decade later, with total catch at 8.6 Mt a year, Japanese vessels found new zones of relatively concentrated activity in waters surrounding New Zealand, off the coast of Southwest Africa, and along Canada's Pacific coast, while fishing with lower intensities was taking place across the entire Indian Ocean, a substantial part of the South Atlantic, and virtually the entire North Pacific.

By 1980 (the harvest in that year was 9.9 Mt) there was some pullback to eastern halves of the Indian and Atlantic Ocean, little change in the Pacific, and a significant extension to the Antarctic waters, where Japan's fishing activities peaked by 1990. Record landings of above 11 Mt took place in 1984 and again during the three successive years between 1986 and 1988. Afterward the trend of Japan's fishing activities shifted rapidly, with 1990 landings at 9.6 Mt, 6.4 Mt in 2000, and only 5.7 Mt in 2007. This decline has been a result of several trends: declining stocks of fish in the Sea of Japan and the nearby Pacific waters; reduced opportunities in distant Pacific, Atlantic, and Indian Ocean regions due to their full exploitation or serious overfishing; rising competition by fishing fleets from China and South Korea; and new fishing fleets of the Pacific island nations. A declining domestic labor force has been yet another reason behind Japan's strong shift toward seafood imports that began during the late 1980s. Seafood imports more than doubled between 1985 and 1995 and have stayed above 3 Mt a year ever since.

Higher imports of aquatic products have not entirely made up for the lower catches by Japan's own fishing fleet, and as a result, the annual per capita supply of seafood (after subtracting nonfood uses and waste) had recorded its first (albeit marginal) postwar decline during the 1990s, from about 70 to about 67 per capita. Even so, Japan retained its position as the world's largest per capita consumer of seafood until the end of the twentieth century, but translating that primacy into reasonably accurate international comparisons highlighting the country's extraordinarily high claim on the overall stocks and diversity of marine food resources is a frustratingly difficult task.

There are no systematic global statistics of fish landings prior to World War II, but Sarhage and Lundbeck (1992) estimated the total at about 10 Mt during the late 1930s. This would mean that the record Japanese prewar catch would have accounted for more than two-fifths of global seafood landings. In contrast to the pre–World War II data absence, the FAO postwar fishing data series begins in 1950 and offers disaggregated global, regional, and national aggregates of seafood catches as well as data disaggregated by major categories (fish, crustaceans, mollusks, and other invertebrates), as well as for major exploited species (FAO 2011e). Easily calculated quotients of Japanese and global catches would indicate that Japan's share of worldwide landings declined from about 20 percent in 1950 to less than 16 percent by 1970, then rose to about 18 percent by 1980, and then its steady decline reduced it to 10 percent by 2000.

Even then, the last share is five times larger than the country's share of the global population, while the differences between Japan's share of seafood supply and its share of world population were seven-fold in 1980 and six-fold in 1960. These indicators, showing Japan's continued exceptionally high claim on marine fish and invertebrates, can be used to argue that throughout the twentieth century Japan had a disproportionately large role in bringing about what is now a generally recognized serious depletion of many marine fish stocks (Clover 2004; Pauly 2009). At the same time, those indicators, although not grossly misleading, cannot be accurate because the widely cited FAO statistics of global seafood production have a substantial (but difficult to narrow down) margin of error and because even Japan, the country whose economic and social statistics are among the world's most reliable, has had some serious problems with underreporting of actual landings and with illegal fish catches.

FAO statistics have never attempted to account for the worldwide extent of illegal (unreported and unregulated) fishing. When Zeller and Pauly (2007) directed a set of studies reconstructing marine fisheries catches for some key regions, they found that the information supplied to the FAO by many countries underestimates their real catch by half or more. The first attempt to estimate the global level of this underreporting was published only in 2009: Agnew et al. (2009) put the worldwide extent of illegal fishing at between 11 and 26 Mt a year, or an average of between 18 and 21 percent as the share of reported catches during five five-year periods prior to 2004, and their best estimates by species group for the years 2000 to 2003 show rates higher than 30 percent (and as high as 60 percent) for salmon, trout, and smelts; 20 to 30 percent for cods, hake, haddock, shrimp, squid, and octopus; and the lowest (less than 10 percent) illegal catches for tuna, flounders, halibut, and sole.

By far the most worrisome example of Japan's illegal fishing has been a two-decade-long period of overfishing of southern bluefin tuna. This long-lasting transgression became known in 2006 as a result of an independent review of catches of southern bluefin tuna: comparisons of commercial logbooks of Japan's longline tuna fishing fleet (previously seen as highly accurate) and tuna sold in Japan's principal fish markets showed that actual catches exceeded the report amount at least twofold, with the most likely aggregate difference of 178,000 tonnes during the two decades and 133,000 tonnes between 1995 and 2004 (Commission for the Conservation of Southern Bluefin Tuna 2006; Polacheck and Davies 2008). This degree of overfishing meant that, for example, in the year 2000, when Japan's reported catch was just over 5,000 tonnes, the actual take was 15,000 tonnes, or as large as the total global reported catch of that species. No wonder New Zealand was "absolutely outraged" at that level of illegal fishing (Commission for the Conservation of Southern Bluefin Tuna 2006, 3) and that Japan accepted the decision to halve its southern bluefin quota for 2007 to 2011 to 3,000 tonnes (Hayashi 2006).

FAO's global fish catch series is also questionable due to its acceptance of exaggerated reports of China's overall catches. Watson and Pauly (2001) showed why those figures have been distorted. The net result of these countervailing realities—actual worldwide catches were lower than the official total because of China's exaggerated claims, but (and perhaps substantially) higher because of illegal and unreported fishing—remains beyond any reliable quantification. While we may not know the real level of seafood exploitation, there is no doubt that during the latter half of the twentieth century, the top-most layers in marine food webs have been seriously depleted by industrial fishing and that the overall biodiversity of ocean life has declined noticeably.

Impact on Marine Biodiversity

Degradation of heavily exploited marine ecosystems is perhaps most convincingly documented by the declining mean trophic level of exploited species, the phenomenon of fishing down marine food webs, with catches of larger, long-lived carnivorous fish decreasing and the shares of short-lived planktivorous fish and invertebrates rising (Pauly et al. 1998; Pauly et al. 2000). But Japan's fishing effort has defied this global trend as it kept targeting large top carnivorous species. In 1960 about 14 percent of Japan's fish landings were the largest piscivorous predators (tunas, swordfish, skipjacks, sharks)—but in the year 2000 the share was up to about 20 percent; similarly, in 1960 all major carnivorous species (adding salmons, cods and mackerels to the above list) accounted for 49 percent of all Japanese fish landings but in the year 2000 their share was up to 56 percent.

A detailed examination of long-term (1958–2003) fishing trends in the Japan Sea also failed to find any evidence of fishing down the sea's marine food web—but expectedly, it indicated stronger fishing pressure on large predatory species ever since the sudden collapse of sardine stocks (for decades the dominant catch in the sea) that followed record catches of the late 1980s (Tian, Kidokoro, and Watanabe 2006). As a result, by 2007 nearly half of the ninety major fisheries in the waters within Japan's exclusive economic zone were seriously depleted and the government formulated plans for the recovery of nearly eighty affected species.

On the global scale this impact has been particularly disproportionate as far as tunas—large, long-lived (ten to twenty years) top predators that are traditionally the most popular and most highly prized of all fish species in Japan—have been concerned. Japanese official statistics put the total catches of all tuna species at about 15,000 tonnes in 1900, rising to more than 60,000 tonnes per year during the 1930s and peaking at more than 80,000 tonnes per year in 1939 and 1940. But Okamoto's (2004) reconstruction of prewar tuna landings indicate that even before 1914, annual catches of skipjack tunas were 30,000 to 50,000 tonnes and that they rose to more than 100,000 tonnes during the late 1930s. This means that Japan's tuna catches accounted for at least 75 to 80 percent and for as much as 90 percent of total pre–World War II global landings, and according to FAO statistics Japanese fishers caught 63 percent of all landed tunas during the 1950s, 54 percent during the 1960s, 37 percent during the 1970s, 30 percent during the 1980s, and 20 percent during the 1990s, giving a cumulative share of about 32 percent of the global tuna landings between 1950 to 2000 (FAO 2011e).

After adding Japan's substantial post-1980 tuna imports and adjusting (conservatively) for unreported overfishing, the country's cumulative share in the global tuna consumption during the second half of the twentieth century rose to more than 40 percent, or more than fifteen times the country's share of the world's population during the same period. Obviously Japanese preference for tunas has had an exceptionally pronounced effect on reducing the biomass and biodiversity of these large marine predators wherever they are found. But the tuna category lumps together species that are still relatively abundant—particularly the Pacific skipjack used in Japan primarily to make *katsuobushi* and consumed elsewhere mainly canned —with those whose fisheries are about to collapse.

Worm et al. (2006) concluded that the rate of fisheries collapses (when the catches drop below 10 percent of the recorded maxima) has been accelerating and by 2003 29 percent of all currently fished species had to be considered as collapsed. Moreover, that study also found that despite substantial increases in fishing effort, cumulative yields across all species and large marine ecosystems had declined by about 13 percent after reaching the maximum in 1994. Not surprisingly, these declines have been most pronounced for the largest predators, tuna, billfish and swordfish. Using the logbook data from Japan's worldwide fishing activities, Worm et al. (2005) demonstrated that between 1950 and 2000, the predator species density showed gradual declines of about 50 percent in both the Atlantic and Indian oceans and about a 25 percent decline in the Pacific.

No large predatory species has been under a greater fishing pressure than the northern bluefin, the most massive (maximum weight in excess of 600 kg, maximum length above 3 meters) of all tunas with a long life span (on the order of twenty years) and warm-blooded metabolism. Its two Atlantic populations (the western, a smaller one, spawning in the Gulf of Mexico and the larger eastern one spawning in the Mediterranean) are particularly endangered. Exploitation of the northern bluefin after World War II began with catches of small fish for canning, but the market changed with Japanese imports of large fish for sushi and *sashimi*, including air deliveries of fresh fish since the early 1970s. As a result, prices rose from a bit more than 10 cents per kg in the late 1960s to about $2.50 per kg by 1975 and to nearly $30 per kg for the fattiest fish by the late 1980s, with the record of $213 per kg for a giant specimen in 1991 (Buck 1995). Since that time, this record has been repeatedly surpassed, and in January 2011, a 342 kg bluefin sold for nearly $396,000, or more than $1,100 per kg (Hosaka 2011); in contrast, yellowfin sells for less than $10 per kg.

Obviously such high prices have led to a common misrepresentation with restaurants mislabeling cheaper tuna meat. An examination of tuna sushi samples from restaurants in New York and Denver indicates frequent instances of such mislabelling (Lowenstein, Amato, and Kolokotronis 2009), and it must be expected that similar practices are found in Japan. More importantly, high *maguro* prices have led to relentless overfishing and declining stocks. Total Atlantic catches rising from the post–World War II low of less than 15,000 tonnes in 1972–1973 to as much as 53,000 tonnes by 1996 and still above 30,000 tonnes since 2000 (International Commission for the Conservation of Atlantic Tunas 2009).

Japan began fishing for the Northern bluefin in 1957 (just 63 t that year) and for the Mediterranean stocks in 1972 (Miyabe 2003) and its total catches were about 4,900 t in 1980, 2,200 t in 1990 and 3,500 t in the year 2000 (about 10 percent of the total). ICCAT's (International Commission for the Conservation of Atlantic Tunas) recent northern bluefin quota of 30,000 tonnes per year was twice the recommended rate based on the best available scientific information—while the actual catch (including underreported and illegal take) has been 50,000 to 60,000 tonnes per year. That is why the World Wildlife Fund has been in the forefront of campaigning for an international trade ban on the Northern bluefin (World Widelife Fund 2010).

This position came to be shared by the fisheries experts of the FAO as well as by the relevant EU governments, and it explains why Monaco had put such a ban on the agenda of the 2010 Convention on International Trade in Endangered Species of Wild Fauna and Flora (CITES). But the proposal, which was strenuously opposed by Japan (which consumes about 80 percent of all Northern tuna) as well as by Canada, China, and South Korea, was defeated on March 18, 2010, by a vote of 20 to 68 (with 30 abstentions). Thus it appears inevitable that without any effective enforcement power, ICCAT will preside over further decline and, very likely, the demise of the fishery (CITES 2010).

The best available information adjusted for unreported overcatch (Miyabe, Miyake, and Nakano 2004; FAO 2011e; Polacheck and Davies 2008; Sonu 2008) indicates that the Japanese landings of bluefin tunas declined from about 75 percent in 1960 to 63 percent by 1980 and about 35 percent by 2000. Japan consumed 45 to 50 percent of all bluefin catches during the 1990s and the share rose to 55 percent by 2005. Not surprisingly, Japanese importers are strongly opposed to any bans on exports. In any case, it may be too late: even a complete ban on fishing in the Mediterranean and in the northeast Atlantic might not prevent an impending collapse of that fishery (Mackenzie, Mosegaard, and Rosenberg 2009).

Seafood versus Other Sources of Animal Protein

Finally, it is instructive to contrast some key environmental impacts of seafood and other sources of animal protein, an exercise that is perhaps best introduced by comparing Japan with the United States. In 2005 America's annual supply of animal foods amounted to 380 kg/capita compared to 173 kg/capita in Japan. Judging by this simple weight comparison, an average American every year consumes animal foods that weigh 2.2 times more than those making up average Japanese dietary supply and hence makes a considerably higher claim on the world's food resources. But the reality is not that simple. A closer look should consider the origin of these foods and the mode and metabolic efficiency of their production.

The most obvious distinction is between foods that do not require the killing of animals (all dairy products and eggs) and those that are produced by killing mammals, birds, fish, or invertebrates, domesticated or wild. America's high output of milk and dairy products (liquid milk equivalent of about 270 kg/capita in 2005) and moderate supply of eggs (about 15 kg/capita) means that about 75 percent of the total weight of its animal foods and about 40 percent of its animal protein does not require killing animals. In contrast, in 2005, the corresponding shares in Japan (with liquid milk supply at about 92 kg and egg availability as nearly 17 kg/capita) were 10 percent lower at, respectively, 63 percent and about 30 percent. A country whose traditional faith enjoins it to spare life thus depends relatively more on killings animals than a country whose dominant religion approves of the human dominion over the animals.

As for the production mode and metabolic efficiency, milk can be produced in sustainable manner (be it largely pasture based or with significant supplementary feeding), with minimized environmental impact and a very low input of plant feeds, including roughages that are indigestible by humans. Overall, it is incontestably the best way to secure high-quality animal protein at the least combined environmental and metabolic cost. Egg production is inherently less (but still relatively fairly) efficient, and although it is often carried in less-than-humane conditions in confinement in crowded cages, it too can be done humanely with free-range birds.

In mass terms, the average (boneless) meat supply was about 83 kg in the United States and only 29 kg in Japan, nearly a three-fold difference. The environmental costs of meat eating are substantial. Because no meat production can ever come close to the efficiency of converting phytomass into milk or eggs and because modern (at least partially feedlot-based) beef production is the most inefficient way to produce animal protein, meat production (as already quantified earlier in this chapter) makes large resource claims in terms of land, water, and fertilizer, and intensive feed monocultures also require high-energy inputs, directly as fuel for machinery and indirectly to make the machines, transport the crops, and synthesize fertilizers, herbicides, and pesticides.

Highly concentrated production facilities present obvious environmental hazards (ranging from the leaching of nitrates to emissions of methane), and they subject the animals to confinement that cannot be classified as either sustainable or humane. Moreover, the westward expansion of America's cattle-based agriculture was a key factor leading to the demise of the continent's enormous herds of wild buffalo during the nineteenth century. But America's current meat-centered agriculture does not result in massive decline of wild species, as does Japan's truly global quest for every imaginable kind of seafood. As irrational as this modern meat-producing system may be, its mass slaughter is confined to domesticated animals, there is no problem with raising new generations, and the production can be based entirely on plant feeds (using supplementary protein feeds derived from waste products of other animals is a modern practice that is both unnecessary and highly undesirable).

In contrast, abundant and sustainable seafood supply faces major challenges in all of these matters: large numbers of other animals are killed alongside the targeted species, natural reproduction of a major exploited species is subject to large fluctuations and sudden collapse, artificial breeding is often very challenging, and all fish species that consumers prefer are carnivorous. *Bycatch* is a specific term for the collateral killing of marine species by modern fishery practices (Alverson et al. 2004). Bycatch is composed of all unwanted marine species that are not targeted by a particular fishery. It is most often other fish species, invertebrates, mammals (most often dolphins), reptiles (most often turtles enmeshed in fishing nets), and sometimes even seabirds, particularly albatrosses and petrels killed by tuna longline fishery (Gales, Brothers, and Reid 1998). But it can also include desirable commercial species that are under the allowable size, are protected in order to sustain sufficient numbers for breeding, are over the permissible catch quota, or are simply not valuable enough in comparison to the principal catch.

Even more unfortunately, some of this collateral killing affects species that are already endangered because of excessive harvesting or changing environmental conditions. Bycatch species are simply discarded over board and both their share in specific fisheries and their survival rates vary widely, which is why there are so few representative larger-scale studies of this phenomenon. The most comprehensive review of bycatch, based on some 800 studies, showed its worldwide mean to be about 35 percent, with specific rates ranging widely: less than 10 percent for cephalopods, more than 60 percent for redfish and bass, 75 percent for flounder and sole, more than 80 percent for eel, nearly 250 percent for crab, to more than 500 percent for shrimp (Alverson et al. 2004). This share translated to about 27 Mt a year for 1990.

A recent detailed analysis of bycatch by small trawlers in the Ariake Sea (the largest bay on the western coast of Kyūshū) indicated a similar rate of about 33 percent (Hirai and Nishinokubi 2004). But there are also indications that thanks to better fishing techniques the global rates of discards have been declining: Alverson (2005) put their total at about 15 (10–20) Mt a year and Kelleher (2004) offered a total as low as 7.3 (6.8–8.0) Mt a year. Given the inherently great variability of these estimates and a truly worldwide sourcing of both Japanese catches and imports, it is impossible to come up with a satisfactory mean discard rate. And the ranges of discard mortality estimates are no smaller, ranging from lows of just a few percent to highs of more than 80 percent or even 100 percent for such species as halibut, king crab, and salmon (Alverson et al. 2004). This means that any assumptions are only illustrative of an important phenomenon and the real values may be substantially different.

When assuming, very conservatively, that bycatch for all of Japan's seafood supply is just 25 percent and that just half of the discarded bycatch does not survive the violent experience, then Japan's overall seafood harvest and imports, totaling 10.2 Mt in 2005, represent aggregate killing of about 11.5 Mt of marine animals, or about 90 kg/capita. In addition, in comparison with the meat supply that is available for domestic consumption, a much smaller share of seafood supply ends up as food. In the first instance, the Japanese share was nearly 65 percent in 2005 (3.6 Mt of 5.6 Mt of meat ended up as food), and in the second, it was only about 43 percent (4.4 Mt of the total of 10.2 Mt). Of course, using the total including dead bycatch would lower the share to less than 40 percent).

Given the many well-documented collapses of major fisheries, little has to be said about the vulnerability of seafood harvests to sudden (and sometimes apparently irreversible) drops in harvest. Artificial breeding is the best way to reduce these risks, but practicing it at reasonable costs and in environmentally acceptable manner is often difficult. Sessile invertebrates (mussels, oysters) are a more manageable choice because of the potentially high density of production and because they have no special feeding needs. In contrast, most fish produced by modern aquaculture in affluent countries are (unlike in China where herbivorous and omnivorous fish dominate) carnivorous species: salmon, seabream, seabass, amberjack, and bluefin tuna must be fed other marine organisms, smaller fish or invertebrates. Expanding mariculture of these carnivores may ease the pressure on their harvesting in wild, but it leads to higher demand for fish protein and fish oil for feeding.

Japan's aquaculture declined from being the world's fourth largest in 2000 to the ninth place by 2007, with recent annual output around 750,000 tonnes, of which two-thirds are shellfish cultures, mainly scallops and oysters, bivalves that filter-feed plankton suspended in the water column. Fish mariculture has been above 200,000 tonnes a year since 1987, and its recent annual means were between 250,000 and 270,000 tonnes. As elsewhere in affluent countries with sizable aquacultures, Japan's marine fish cultures are dominated by carnivorous species, with the largest landings coming from yellowtails (around 150,000 tonnes per year) and red sea bream (about 80,000 tonnes per year), followed by greater amberjack (*kanpachi*), olive flounder (*hirame*), *fugu,* and jack mackerel (*aji*). Their production needs more than 2 Mt (fresh weight) of fish feeds annually to provide the necessary protein and fish oils.

This brief comparison of two very different modes of securing plentiful supplies of animal protein ends up with surprisingly similar conclusions. America's excessive red meat and poultry consumption cannot be extended to the rest of the world. The U.S. population is less than 5 percent of the world total, but it consumes nearly 15 percent of all meat produced by feeding domesticated animals. If a similar level of consumption were to be replicated worldwide, there would not be enough high-quality feed (corn and soybeans) to produce so much poultry, pork, and beef; moreover, the requisite energy needs would tax the global supply of hydrocarbons even further, combustion of these fuels would increase emissions of CO_2, and larger ruminant herds would produce more CH_4. High levels of meat intake would be problematic even if the environmental impacts of intensive animal husbandry were kept to a minimum: international comparisons indicate that high levels of carnivory contribute to high rates of overweight, obesity, and several chronic diseases.

Japan's claim on marine protein is relatively even greater than America's claim on terrestrial meat protein: the country with not even 2 percent of the world's population now consumes more than 8 percent of all seafood, and it cannot be—all the talk about the nutritional desirability of eating fish aside—a model for populous modernizing nations because all major fishing regions are either already overfished or harvested very close to their sustainable capacity. Japan and the United States, whose foodways differ in so many important ways, share an important, and unenviable, commonality: both have overreached in their quest for animal protein, and their consumption cannot be models for those modernizing countries that rightly aspire to higher intakes of high-quality animal protein.

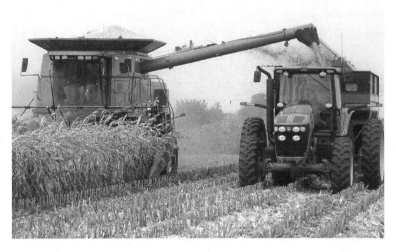

Harvesting corn in Iowa: most of Japan's food now originates abroad, with U.S. feed corn being the single largest annual import in terms of mass. (Iowa State University)

6

Japanese Diet: Retrospect and Prospect

Fascination of long-term perspectives lies in dynamic combinations of gradual trends, which often unfold in unpredictable ways, and sudden shifts whose power sets entire nations on new historical trajectories. The history of modern Japan is a near-perfect example of this interaction. The five generations of a deliberate, underlying trend of economic, technical, and social modernization, which began with the fall of last Tokugawa *shōgun* in 1867, were punctuated by events that redefined the nation's future course. None of these were more important than the decision to attack the United States in December 1941 and the resulting military defeat in August 1945.

The defeat had consequences that could not have been anticipated during the autumn of 1945, when economically prostrate Japan, barely able to feed itself, began reconstruction. After the country regained its prewar economic standing, the overall pace of its change intensified, and less than four decades later, during the late 1980s, it was not only the world's second largest economy (in aggregate terms) but also one of the most affluent (in per capita terms) and one widely perceived to become even more successful in the century's last decade and far beyond. Once again, nobody could have anticipated in 1990, when Japan's economic miracle began to fall apart, that there will be no clear end to this great unraveling even two decades later.

Not surprisingly, Japan's dietary transition has mirrored these great trends and shifts: deliberate, gradual, but relatively still fairly slow changes of the first Meiji decades, their post–World War I intensification that ended with the attack on the United States, admirable gains during the four postwar decades in general, and between the late 1960s and the late 1980s in particular, the great post-1990 dénouement that led to new realities of an economically stagnant Japan whose population is not only aging at a rapid rate but it is also to soon begin a long trend of absolute decline. As a result, new concerns have emerged, perhaps none of them more prominent than Japan's low degree of self-sufficiency in agricultural production and the supply of seafood. As always, any specific long-term predictions are bound to be wrong: the best we can do when looking ahead is to outline some major unfolding trends.

A Century of Dietary Transitions

A century ago, Japan was in the fifth decade of its modernization that began with the formal restoration of the imperial power in February 1867 and eventually progressed to an elected parliament and, after a quarter millennium of self-imposed isolation, a forceful entry into foreign affairs. Its industrial base, overall economic might, and military capacity were rapidly expanding, but the typical diet of its citizens, and particularly the majority people still living in rural areas, was not fundamentally different qualitatively and quantitatively from the nutrition available during the last decades of the Tokugawa *shōgun* rule. Rice was the most important grain, but everyday diets contained a great deal of less desirable coarse cereals; large segments of the population ate virtually no animal foods; the selection of vegetables and fruits was limited; and average food energy intakes were barely adequate to cover basic metabolic and activity needs, resulting in widespread stunted growth.

Some important gains took place between the two world wars: extension of the North Pacific fisheries (particularly the catches of skipjack, *katsuo*) and the launching of first long-distance fishing vessels, rising rice and sugar imports from Korea and Taiwan (Japan's two Asian colonies), a slow expansion of dairy production, and, among urban elites, new tastes for coffee, black tea, Western alcoholic beverages, and cakes and other sweets. But the shifts in terms of average food supply and consumption were slow and limited, and all interwar gains were erased by Japan's defeat in World War II. It took a decade after the war to surpass the average per capita peak prewar food supply but its subsequent progress was rapid, driven by decades of rapid economic growth.

Japan's dietary transition made its greatest advances during the three decades between the mid-1950s and the mid-1980s. Most of its changes followed a universal transition pattern: falling intakes of carbohydrates in general and of rice, the dominant staple grain, in particular; lower consumption of legumes and tubers; higher consumption of fruits and all kinds of animal foodstuffs, including previously very low consumption of meat (with pork in the lead) and virtually nonexistent consumption of milk and other dairy products. And contrary to a common impression, average fish consumption remained relatively low before World War II; it rose to a level unparalleled worldwide only during the 1960s. Other dietary changes with common counterparts in other modernizing nations included higher consumption of cooking oils, more sugar, more alcoholic beverages, a rapid adoption of coffee and soft drinks, a much increased consumption of processed foods, and more frequent eating outside the home.

But Japan's dietary transition has also had some specific features that have kept the country's typical food consumption distinct. In terms of individual foodstuffs, these have included continued relatively high consumption of soybean-based foods (tofu, *miso*, *shōyu*), raw fish (with sushi as an unexpected culinary export), preference for tuna species as both the basic and the most prized seafood (skipjack for *katsuobushi* to make the ubiquitous soup stock and *maguro* for the costliest *nigirizushi*), demand for perfect looking vegetables and fruit, and continued fondness for green tea and sweets based on bean paste (*anko*). In terms of macro- and micronutrients, it is necessary to note surprisingly limited increases in intakes of fat (with the lowest shares of lipid energy among affluent nations) and simple carbohydrates (sugar and other sweeteners) and continued high intakes of salt.

The diet that has emerged from this transition presents a remarkable fusion of different culinary traditions. Its ancient foundation is a combination of classic Chinese ingredients with many modifications introduced during more than a millennium of the evolution of Japan's indigenous cuisine; its modern transformation has been heavily influenced by a wide variety of both traditional and modern European and American food choices, some adopted intact and many altered to suit Japanese preferences. Visually there is no better confirmation of this fusion than a visit to a modern Japanese supermarket, with its rich choice of traditional Japanese foodstuffs alongside a seemingly no smaller choice of Western ingredients.

Statistically there is perhaps no better indicator of the westernization of the modern Japanese diet than the size of the country's ten largest food processors (ranked by net sales). Four of them are primarily brewers of beer and distillers of liquors (Asahi, Kirin, and Suntory are the three top ones; Sapporo Holdings is number eight), two are in the dairy business (Meiji Dairies and Morinaga Milk Industry, numbers nine and ten), one is a meat packer (Nippon, number six), and one is a baker (Yamazaki, number seven). Maruha Group, the country's largest marine product company, the fourth in overall net sales, and Ajinomoto, number five, complete the group (Aoki 2007).

Perhaps the most notable characteristic of Japan's dietary transition has been its overall restraint. As the quality and variety of Japanese diets have improved considerably, the average per capita supply of food energy has stayed as much as 1,000 kcal a day lower than in many Western nations, and the average intakes, after rising well above 2,000 kcal a day, moved (with aging and decreased physical activity) below 1,900 kcal a day. This dietary restraint has certainly been a major reason for Japan's very low obesity rate, and it has played an important role in the nation's record-breaking life expectancy. But, not surprisingly, nutritional specifics behind this accomplishment have not been easy to isolate. Is it high seafood intake, habitual drinking of green tea, plenty of soy foods, or all of the above (and other, nondietary, factors) that foster the country's longevity?

What is easier to do is to note several considerable environmental impacts of Japan's dietary transition, both domestically and abroad. High domestic rice yields supported by high applications of nitrogenous fertilizers and increasing concentrations of domestic animals have burdened Japan's water with excessive amounts of reactive nitrogen. Large imports of many food and feed crops (grains, soybeans, oil seeds, vegetables, and fruits) mean that the country's food supply now claims more farmland, more water, and more fertilizer in the exporting countries (above all in the United States, Canada, Brazil, and China) than it does in Japan. Japan's very high fish consumption has caused a serious decline of most of the fisheries along the country's coasts and within its economic zone, and rising seafood imports have been a major factor contributing to the worldwide loss of marine biodiversity, a concern that is particularly acute as far as the most valuable tuna stocks are concerned.

But when seen from the domestic Japanese perspective, these matters are overshadowed by a simpler and more immediate concern: What are the current and, more so, future implications of the country's high dependence on food imports? Does this dependence compromise its long-term physical well-being and security? If so, are there any realistic steps whose committed pursuit could increase Japan's food self-sufficiency? These are understandable concerns that are subject to emotional judgments and hence can be easily exaggerated, but because there are no perfect measures of self-sufficiency and no clear demarcations between the feeling of security and worries about excessive dependence, it is much more difficult to offer a dispassionate analysis of the self-sufficiency challenge.

Concerns about Japan's Food Self-Sufficiency

As this book makes clear, Japan enjoys a rich, varied, and healthy diet, and it does not have to spend extravagantly to import what it cannot, or prefers not to, harvest or produce. In 2008 foreign food accounted for 10.6 percent of the total value of Japan's imports. For comparison, the shares were (as expected) significantly lower for the world's two major food producers, the United States and Canada (at, respectively, 5.3 and 7.5 percent), but in 2008, food accounted for 9.6 percent of the European Union's imports (World Trade Organization 2010). Moreover, Japan's total bill for foreign food came to about $80 billion, an equivalent of only about 10 percent of its export earnings, while Americans spent an equivalent of 9 percent of their exports on food and the EU paid 10.3 percent. These comparisons do not show any exceptional Japanese exposure and do not indicate that the country is intolerably dependent on foreign foods and should feel insecure.

And increasing food imports have not resulted in any catastrophic long-term financial burdens. In 1975 the total value of Japanese food imports was equal to only 17 percent of the nation's food supply, and by 2000 it rose to 29 percent. Expressed in inverse terms, Japan's food self-sufficiency fell from 83 percent in 1975 to 71 percent by 2000. All of these facts would hardly be panic inducing, but if a domestic policy goal is to promote agricultural production—and to make the population less anxious about the dependence on imported food—then another measure can convey the same situation in a suitably worrisome manner. And that is precisely why Japanese policymakers decided to express the country's food self-sufficiency ratio not in financial terms but as a "calorie ratio," a quotient of domestically produced food energy and the total food energy supply that shows a far greater deterioration than does the monetary comparison

Because of Japan's rising post-1960 dependence on imports of food-stuffs with relatively high energy density (corn, soybeans, meat), this ratio was declining for the last four decades of the twentieth century, from about 73 percent in 1960 to 54 percent by 1975 and 40 percent by 2000; subsequently, it held steady at 40 percent, fell to 39 percent in 2006, recovered again to 40 percent or slightly higher for the next three years, but fell again to 39 percent in 2010. Recently the individual components of the ratio have ranged from highs of 95-97 percent for rice and sweet potatoes to about 80 percent for vegetables, to only 26-33 percent for sugar, 5 percent for soybeans, and 2 percent for plant oils (Ministry of Agriculture, Forests and Fisheries 2010). In addition, most of Japan's meat production depends on feed imports from other countries, most notably the United States. For example, about 90 percent of all concentrate feed must be imported, and the country has to buy even a significant part of roughage feed (about 25 percent) abroad. When domestic animal food production based on imported feed (expressed in total digestible nutrients) is counted as foreign based, the self-sufficiency of animal foodstuffs drops to only about 15 percent as of 2009. This high dependence makes a major contribution to the less than 50 percent food self-sufficiency on an energy basis.

The ratio's long fall and its slippage below 50 percent (and temporarily even below 40 percent) has become a chronic worry for Japanese policymakers who have turned food self-sufficiency (*shokuryō jikyū ritsu*) into a major national concern. Official Japanese publications, echoed by media reports, stress that no other affluent country is so dangerously dependent on food imports, and they compare the country's low self-sufficiency ratio with much higher shares for the United States, Canada, and France (all being major agricultural exporters with ratios well above 100 percent), Germany (above 80 percent), Britain (about 70 percent), and Switzerland (at nearly 60 percent).

And the government—trying to defy the rapid aging of Japan's agricultural and fishery labor force and in disregard of very high costs and some relatively low productivities of domestic food production—has been trying to reverse the trend. In March 2000 it set a target of 45 percent food self-sufficiency by the year 2010—but before long, it was forced to postpone the target date to 2015. Some specific targets included meaningless increases for crops that can be produced much more profitably and with less environmental impact abroad: a 2 percent boost for soybeans (from 3 to 5 percent) and a 3 percent gain for wheat (from 9 to 12 percent).

Moreover, in April 2008 the Ministry of Agriculture, Forestry, and Fisheries (MAFF) set up the new Food Security Department (whose mission is to increase public awareness of what the ministry labels "the country's poor food self-sufficiency rate"), and in October 2008 it launched Food Action Nippon (*Fūdo akushon nippon*) , a campaign whose Web site (with its animal cartoons and a logo that shows a smiley-like face about to bite into a red circle, an enticement to eat jam made with rice flour) has garnered many celebrity endorsements as it aims to create a massive social network to support the aims of higher food self-sufficiency (Syokuryo 2010). This strategy has worked: a January 2009 poll indicated that 91 percent of respondents thought that Japan should increase its food self-sufficiency rate and about 72 percent claimed that they are "consciously" or "very consciously" trying to eat domestic food (Japan for Sustainability 2009).

In December 2008, in the wake of significant food price spikes, MAFF began to propose a 50 percent food self-sufficiency share by 2017 to be accomplished by increasing average per capita rice consumption by 2 kg, raising rice flour and feed rice production, doubling wheat harvest, and more than doubling soybean output. And Mashimo (2008), in a study prepared for the Consumers Union of Japan, went even further, suggesting (quite unrealistically) that by changing diets, planting more than 2 Mha of land, in addition to the cultivated area in 2005, and raising domestic yield, it could be possible to increase food self-sufficiency to the range of 75 to 80 percent.

At the same time, it is obvious that food energy self-sufficiency ratios are to a large extent arbitrary indicators that provide little information about the actual security of the food supply or the quality of available nutrition. A poor and still largely agricultural economy with a barely adequate food supply can have high self-sufficiency ratio for its staple grain, and Canada's seafood self-sufficiency ratio (above 125 percent) is among the highest worldwide because Canadian fish consumption is relatively low (lower than in most Western European countries). Yet many expensive imports that make little difference to overall nutrition (ranging from shrimp to tropical fruits) and may significantly contribute to higher import ratios could decline with a minimal impact in a more frugal economic climate.

Even so, the reasons for concern about rising shares of food, both raw and processed, coming from foreign countries are understandable. The first one is the magnitude of dependence: Japan's imports are disproportionately large in relation to its population (less than 2 percent of the world total). The country has been the world's largest importer of cereal grains and meat (accounting for just over 8 percent of respective global sales in 2008), and only in 2007 were its seafood imports narrowly surpassed by those of the United States. Perhaps the most important personal concern is about the safety of imported food. This became a particularly contentious matter in 2008, when many Japanese consumers became sick after eating pesticide-contaminated *gyōza* imported from China. In a nationwide survey in early February 2008, 75 percent of respondents said they will not eat Chinese food, an impractical resolution given the magnitude of Japan's food imports from China.

In 2008 large price increases for energy, food, and fertilizer also focused attention on Japan's vulnerability to sudden price spikes, caused by inclement weather in exporting countries or rising cost of energy and fertilizer, and had intensified the lingering concerns about the rising demand for food imports in rapidly industrializing populous countries that will lead to greater global price competition and a possible loss of purchases to other buyers (the event known as *kaimake*). And there are also worries about the environmental impacts of intercontinental food transportation, above all about the energy needed to do that and resulting greenhouse gas emissions.

But none of these understandable concerns need to be feared obstacles to Japan's comfortable dependence on food imports. A high level of dependence on imported commodities is common in the global economy, and going back to high levels of economic autarky is both impractical and undesirable. Many affluent nations now buy large shares (often more than 90 percent) of their energy (particularly crude oil), mineral ores, metals, chemicals, fertilizers, and manufactures (ranging from toys to cars) abroad, and they do not need to be concerned about it as long as the value of their imports is at least balanced or even surpassed by the value of their exports (Japan being a prime example of the latter case).

Worries about food safety can be eased by stronger bilateral and international agreements. Price spikes in the global economy are not limited to importers (be they of oil or wheat): Canada exports both oil and wheat, and when their prices spiked in 2008 Canadian consumers were not exempt from the impact. Economic modernization in Asia and Latin America has increased demand for many commodities, but during the past generation, there have been no large or persistent gaps in food available for foreign sale.

Careful studies show that in many cases, the simplistic "food miles" concept cannot withstand critical examination. Concerns about the energy and environmental costs of long-distance shipments have been a leading factor behind the advocacy of locally produced and locally consumed food. *Chisan-chishō*, the Japanese version of this fashionable movement, which began as a quest for slow food during the late 1980s in Europe (Portinari et al. 1989) and now has many promoters in affluent countries, has been active since the late 1990s (Kimura and Nishiyama 2008). But a closer look shows that this is actually a minor burden. Japan's food imports were estimated to require about 900 billion tonne-kilometers per year, an average distance of 15,000 km per shipment (Nakata 2003). Even when assuming an average energy cost of shipping at 200 kilojoules per tonne-kilometer this would translate to an equivalent of about 4.3 Mt of crude oil, or less than 2 percent of Japan's oil consumption and just 0.8 percent of its primary energy use, hardly an intolerably high figure and a total that could be reduced or easily saved by other efficiency adjustments.

Moreover, expressing the burden by linear distance between a producer and consumer ignores the often much higher productivity of growing the food in a distant but optimally endowed place as well as the efficiency of modern marine transportation systems (be they bulk dry-cargo carriers moving grains or refrigerated containers on massive ships used to export meat and dairy foods). As a result, an ideologically preconceived preference for local food (and policies promoting its adoption) may result in higher overall energy needs and greater emissions of greenhouse gases (Desrochers and Shimizu 2009; Capper, Cady, and Bauman 2009). And in any case, there are more fundamental factors that will make it very difficult (and most likely impossible) for Japan to alter its recent food supply pattern.

Long-Term Outlook

We have looked at a century of Japan's dietary transition, but nobody can say anything convincing about where the country, and the rest of the world, will be at the close of the twenty-first century. Despite the increasing popularity of long-range forecasts, all attempts that range further than two generations are just fairy tales (some boring, some provocative). A generational outlook, twenty to thirty years ahead, rests on a firmer ground because most of the mothers of that new generation are already with us, as are most urban, industrial, and transportation infrastructures and institutional arrangements. In Japan's case, the combination of aging and declining population will exert a particularly strong effect on the country's food regime during the coming three decades.

Population projections anticipate the total population declining from nearly 127 million in 2010 to about 117 million by 2030 and just below 110 million by 2040, with an annual loss of more than 700,000 during the 2030s (United Nations 2008). Concurrently, the median age will rise from 44.7 to 54.4 years and by 2040, there will be nearly 30 percent more people aged 80 and above than children up to 14 years of age. This will be the first time in human history that octogenerians will outnumber children. People will also live longer: by 2040 life expectancy will be 82.6 years for males and 90.0 years for females, and there will be nearly half a million Japanese aged 100 or more years.

That will be a problematic achievement. As a study of the functional status of centenarians in Tokyo showed, only 18 percent could be classified as normal, with 55 percent being frail (with impairment of either cognitive or physical functions) and 25 percent fragile, exhibiting both mental and physical deterioration (Gondo et al. 2006). Multiplying this half a million times does not make for a comforting prospect. Other implications of these demographic trends are clear, and they could be reversed only by allowing a relatively high and continuous level of immigration or by an unprecedented rebound of fertility. Both of these developments are highly unlikely.

Overall food demand will remain fairly stable or it will be slightly declining during the next few years, and the decline will accelerate during the 2020s as average per capita intakes will keep falling further below 2,000 kcal a day as daily energy expenditures of many elderly people will fall below 1,500 kcal a day. A combination of several demographic, social, and economic factors makes it almost inevitable that Japan's domestic capacity to feed itself will decline further, and imports will have to fill an even higher share of consumption. Aging of the agricultural labor force has been relentless, and it will only accelerate. In 1990 32 percent of all male farmers were older than 65 years, and by 2008, that ratio had surpassed 60 percent (Statistics Bureau 2011b). Shrinking numbers of fishermen (they fell by more than 25 percent between 1997 and 2007) will be aggravated by the fact that fewer than 20 percent of today's fishery workers have a successor for their job (Ministry of Agriculture, Forestry, and Fisheries 2008b). Long-lasting decline of cultivated land (there was a 13 percent decline between 1988 and 2008) and a greater global competition for seafood will add to the demographic problems.

What is less clear is the impact of aging on specific food demand. Some believe that the aging of the population will result in at least a partial comeback of the traditional diet, with less meat and more vegetables, fruits, and fish (Bittencourt, Teratanavat, and Chern 2007). But that looks increasingly like wishful thinking: the post-1995 consumption data indicate what the MAFF (2006) called an unprecedented "shift away from fish." Average daily per capita intakes of meat and fish had been converging for many years, and in 2006 meat edged out fish for the first time. And while people aged 59 and above still buy about 20 kg of fresh fish per capita every year, the average rate fell to only 5 kg for people younger than 30 years old, similar to typical purchases in many EU countries.

Moreover, public opinion surveys show that 56 percent of all people eat more meat than fish as their main dish, 62 percent prefer meat while eating out, and 65 percent prefer meat when consuming ready-to-eat meals at home (Ministry of Agriculture, Forestry, and Fisheries 2006). The most common reasons are that some family members dislike fish (about 30 percent), fish is more expensive than meat (another 30 percent), and cooking fish is bothersome (about 25 percent). As a result, it appears that before too long (perhaps as early as 2015), the average fish consumption will be back to where it was in 1970 before it rose steadily during the 1970s, 1980s, and 1990s. Even more important, 70 percent of women in their 30s do not cook fish—and their main reason is that less than 50 percent of children like it (Ministry of Agriculture, Forestry, and Fisheries 2008b), a potent indicator of further long-term decline in seafood consumption. As for rice, it is most unlikely that promotion of such nontraditional foodstuffs as germinated brown rice and rice bread or diffusion of drive-through *onigiri* dispensers are going to reverse the long-term decline in rice consumption: the best that can be hoped for is a slower rate of decrease, or even a temporary stabilization.

But all such particulars are merely consequences created by the underlying historical trends or sudden shifts. The primary driver of Japan's future food supply and consumption will be, as it has been during the past century, the overall strength of the country's economy and the capacity to meet difficult long-term challenges. For eight decades after its reopening to the rest of the world, Japan was successful, although not spectacularly so, on both accounts; afterward it overreached with its military aggression, but then it found new purpose and met new challenges during the decades of its widely admired postwar economic and social progress. In 1990 everything began to change once again, and two decades later there is still no discernible end to this period of underperformance, decline, and doubts.

But Japan, arguably more than other ancient nations with a successful record of modernization, is a country intimately aware of the impermanence of things (*mujō*), and this also means that while its future will be influenced by its current economic difficulties and circumscribed by its demographic realities, it is not preordained by either its complex past or its sobering present. Only in retrospect will we be able to judge the real extent and the consequences of the coming economic and social changes— and of Japan's fascinating food transition, now in its second century.

References

Agnew, D. J., et al. 2009. Estimating the worldwide extent of illegal fishing. *PLoS ONE* 4 (2):e4570. doi:10.1371/journal.pone.0004570.

Ajinomoto. 2010. Ajinomoto Corporation. 味の素株式会社 [*Ajinomoto kabushiki kaisha*]. http://www.ajinomoto.com

Allan, J. A. 1993. Fortunately there are substitutes for water otherwise our hydropolitical futures would be impossible. In *Priorities for Water Resources Allocation and Management*, 13–26. London: ODA.

Allen, R. G., et al. 1998. *Crop Evapotranspiration*. Rome: Food and Agriculture Organization.

Alverson, D. L. 2005. Managing the catch of non-target species. In *Improving Fishery Management: Melding Science and Governance*, ed. W. S. Wooster and J. M. Quinn. Seattle: School of Marine Affairs, University of Washington.

Alverson, D. L., et al. 2004. *A Global Assessment of Fisheries Bycatch and Discards*. Rome: Food and Agriculture Organization.

American Soybean Association. 2009. Grower opportunities for identity preserved value-added soybeans. http://www.soygrowers.com/ipvas

Aoki, S. T. 2007. *Japan Food Processing Ingredients Sector; Japanese Food Processing Sector*. Tokyo: U.S. Department of Agriculture, Foreign Agricultural Service. http://www.fas.usda.gov/gainfiles/200703/146280587.pdf

Arimoto, Y. 2010. *Simply Japanese: Modern Cooking for the Healthy Home*. New York: Kodansha International.

Ashkenazi, M., and J. Jacob. 2000. *The Essence of Japanese Cuisine: An Essay on Food and Culture*. Philadelphia: University of Pennsylvania Press.

Attarod, P., M. Aoki, and V. Bayramzadeh. 2009. Measurements of the actual evapotranspiration and crop coefficients of summer and winter seasons crops in Japan. *Plant, Soil and Environment* 55:121–127.

Australian Seafood Cooperative Research Center. 2009. Historical breakthrough in tuna aquaculture. http://www.pir.sa.gov.au/__data/assets/pdf_file/0007/109366/HISTORICAL_BREAKTHROUGH_IN_TUNA_AQUACULTURE.pdf

Bassino, J. 2006. The growth of agricultural output, and food supply in Meiji Japan: Economic miracle or statistical artifact? *Economic Development and Cultural Change* 54:503–521.

Becker, G. S. 2005. *Japan-U.S. Beef Trade Issues.* Washington, DC: Congressional Research Service. http://www.nationalaglawcenter.org/assets/crs/RS22115.pdf

Bengoa, J. M. 2001. Food transition in the twentieth–twenty-first century. *Public Health Nutrition* 4 (6A):1425–1427.

Benihana. 2010. Benihana menu. http://www.benihana.com/menu

Bergin, A., and M. Haward. 1996. *Japan's Tuna Fishing Industry: A Setting Sun or New Dawn?* Commack, NY: Nova Science Publishers.

Bestor, T. C. 2004. *Tsukiji: The Fish Market at the Center of the World.* Berkeley: University of California Press.

Bittencourt, M. V. L., R. P. Tetratanavat, and W. S. Chern. 2007. Food consumption and demographics in Japan: Implications for an aging population. *Agribusiness* 23:529–551.

Buck, E. H. 1995. *Atlantic Bluefin Tuna: International Management of a Shared Resource.* CRS Report for Congress. Washington, DC: U.S. Congress.

Business Wire. 2006. Hawaii's Kona deep deep sea drinking water becomes national brand in Japan. http://www.allbusiness.com/services/business-services/3972264-1.html

Caballero, B., and B. M. Popkin, eds. 2002. *The Nutrition Transition: Diet and Disease in the Developing World.* Amsterdam: Academic Press.

Campo, I. S., and J. C. Beghin. 2005. *Dairy Food Consumption, Production, and Policy in Japan.* Ames: Center for Agricultural and Rural Development, Iowa State University.

Capper, J. L., R. A. Cady, and D. E. Bauman. 2009. Demystifying the environmental sustainability of food production. In *Proceedings of the Cornell Nutrition Conference 2009.* Ithaca, NY: Cornell University. http://wsu.academia.edu/documents/0046/7264/2009_Cornell_Nutrition_Conference_Capper_et_al.pdf

Caprio, M., and Y. Sugita. 2007. *Democracy in Occupied Japan: The U.S. Occupation and Japanese Politics and Society.* London: Routledge.

Carpenter, K. J. 2000. *Beriberi, White Rice, and Vitamin B: A Disease, a Cause, and a Cure.* Berkeley: University of California Press.

Centers for Disease Control. 2004. Trends in intake of energy and macronutrients—United States, 1971–2000. http://www.cdc.gov/mmwr/preview/mmwrhtml/mm5304a3.htm

Chamberlain, B. H. 1890. *Japanese Things.* Tokyo: Hakubunsha.

Chang, S. T., and P. G. Miles. 2004. *Mushrooms: Cultivation, Nutritional Value, Medicinal Effect, and Environmental Impact.* Boca Raton, FL: CRC Press.

Chapagain, A. K., and A. Y. Hoekstra. 2004. *Main Report.* vol. 1. *Water Footprints of Nations.* Paris: UNESCO-IHE.

Chapple, C. 1993. *Nonviolence to Animals, Earth and Self in Asian Traditions.* Albany: State University of New York Press.

Chern, W. S., et al. 2003. *Analysis of the Food Consumption of Japanese Households.* Rome: Food and Agriculture Association.

Clapham, P. J., et al. 2007. The whaling issue: Conservation, confusion, and casuistry. *Marine Policy* 31:314–319.

Clement, Y. 2009. Can green tea do that? A literature review of the clinical evidence. *Preventive Medicine* 49:83–87.

Clover, C. 2004. *The End of Line: How Over-Fishing Is Changing the World and What We Eat*. London: Ebury Press.

Commission for the Conservation of Southern Bluefin Tuna. 2006. *Report of the Special Meeting of the Extended Commission; Appendix 3*. http://www.ccsbt.org/docs/meeting_r.html

Conlon, M. 2009a. *The History of U.S. Soybean Exports to Japan*. Tokyo: U.S. Department of Agriculture, Foreign Agricultural Service. http://www.fas.usda.gov/itp/Japan/JA9502SoybeanExports012309FINAL.pdf

Conlon, M. 2009b. *The History of U.S. Beef and Pork Exports to Japan*. Tokyo: U.S. Department of Agriculture, Foreign Agricultural Service. http://www.usdajapan.org/en/reports/History%20of%20US%20Beef%20and%20Pork.pdf

Convention on International Trade in Endangered Species of Wild Fauna and Flora. 2010. Governments not ready for trade ban on bluefin tuna. http://www.cites.org/eng/news/press_release.shtml

Corkeron, P. J. 2009. Reconsidering the science of scientific whaling. *Marine Ecology Progress* 375:305–309.

Cwiertka, K. J. 2007. *Modern Japanese Cuisine: Food, Power and National Identity*. London: Reaktion Books.

Davidson, A. 1999. *The Oxford Companion to Food*. New York: Oxford University Press.

de Datta, S. K., and W. H. Patrick, eds. 1983. *Nitrogen Economy of Flooded Rice Soils*. Dordrecht: M. Nijhoff.

de Fraiture, C., et al. 2004. *Does International Cereal Trade Save Water? The Impact of Virtual Water Trade on Global Water Use*. Colombo: Comprehensive Assessment Secretariat. http://www.iwmi.cgiar.org/Assessment/files/pdf/publications/ResearchReports/CARR4.pdf

Deschamp, V. 1911. The soy bean. *Journal of Agriculture* 9:621–629.

Desrochers, P., and H. Shimizu. 2008. *Yes, We Have No Bananas: Critique of the "Food Miles" Perspective*. Fairfax, VA: George Mason University. http://mercatus.org/sites/default/files/publication/Yes_We_Have_No_Bananas__A_Critique_of_the_Food_Mile_Perspective.pdf

Dore, R. P. 1958. *City Life in Japan*. Berkeley: University of California Press.

Drew, K. M. 1949. *Conchocelis*-phase in the life-history of *Porphyra umbilicalis* (L.) Kütz. *Nature* 164:748–749.

Dunn, C. J. 1969. *Everyday Life in Traditional Japan*. Tokyo: Tuttle Publishing.

Ekuan, K. 1998. *The Aesthetics of the Japanese Lunchbox*. Cambridge, MA: MIT Press.

Endo, T., et al. 2005. Total mercury, methyl mercury, and selenium levels in the red meat of small cetaceans sold for human consumption in Japan. *Environmental Science and Technology* 39:5703–5708.

Espenshade, A. 1949. A program for Japanese fisheries. *Geographical Review* 39:76–85.

Euromonitor International. 2009. *Coffee in Japan*. London: Euromonitor International.

Eurostat. 2011. Final consumption expenditure of households, by consumption purpose. http://epp.eurostat.ec.europa.eu/portal/page/portal/eurostat/home

Ferrières, J. 2004. The French paradox: Lessons for other countries. *Heart (British Cardiac Society)* 90:107–111.

Francks, P. 1984. *Technology and Agricultural Development in Pre-War Japan*. New Haven, CT: Yale University Press.

Francks, P. 2009. Inconspicuous consumption: Sake, beer, and the birth of the consumer in Japan. *Journal of Asian Studies* 68:135–164.

Food and Agriculture Organization. 1959. *Trade Yearbook*. Rome: Food and Agriculture Association.

Food and Agriculture Association. 2011a. Food balance sheets. http://faostat.fao.org/site/368/default.aspx#ancor

Food and Agriculture Association. 2011b. Land use database. http://faostat.fao.org/site/377/default.aspx#ancor

Food and Agriculture Association. 2011c. TradeSTAT. http://faostat.fao.org/site/406/default.aspx

Food and Agriculture Association. 2011d. Aquastat: Global information system on water and agriculture. http://www.fao.org/nr/water/aquastat/countries/index.stm

Food and Agriculture Association. 2011e. Fisheries and Aquaculture Department. http://www.fao.org/fishery/statistics/en

Food and Agriculture Association/World Health Organization. 1993. *Energy and Protein Requirements: Report of a Joint FAO/WHO Ad Hoc Expert Committee*. Rome: FAO.

Fuess, H. 2003. Der Aufbau der Bierindustrie in Japan während der Meiji-Zeit: Konsum, Kapital und Kompetenz. [The origins of the beer industry during the Meiji period: Consumption, capitalism, and competencies] *Bochumer Jahrbuch für Ostasienforschung* 27:231–267.

Fukushima, H. 2007. Toward reduction of environmental burden caused by excessive application of nitrogen fertilizer. *Quarterly Review* 23:23–28.

Fukushima, Y., et al. 2009. Coffee and green tea as a large source of antioxidant polyphenols in the Japanese population. *Journal of Agricultural and Food Chemistry* 57:1253–1259.

Gales, R., N. Brothers, and T. Reid. 1998. Seabird mortality in the Japanese tuna longline fishery around Australia, 1988–1995. *Biological Conservation* 86:37–56.

Galloway, J. N., et al. 2007. International trade in meat: The tip of the pork chop. *Ambio* 36:622–629.

Garby, L. 1990. Metabolic adaptation to decreases in energy intake due to changes in the energy cost of low energy expenditure regimen. *World Review of Nutrition and Dietetics* 61:173–208.

Gauntner, J. 2002. *The Saké Handbook.* Tokyo: Tuttle Publishing.

Geha, R. S., et al. 2000. Review of alleged reaction to monosodium glutamate and outcome of a multicenter double-blind placebo-controlled study. *Journal of Nutrition* 130:1058S–1062S.

Gillett, R. 2007. *A Short History of Industrial Fishing in the Pacific Islands.* Bangkok: Asia-Pacific Fishery Commission.

Global Agriculture Information Network. 2010. Japan food trends. http://www .fas.usda.gov/scriptsw/AttacheRep/attache_lout.asp

Gondo, Y., et al. 2006. Functional status of centenarians in Tokyo, Japan: Developing better phenotypes of exceptional longevity. *Journals of Gerontology. Series A, Biological Sciences and Medical Sciences* 61:305–310.

GOO. 2007. Ranking foods after returning from a trip abroad. http://ranking .goo.ne.jp/ranking/013/gethome_food

Gortner, W. A. 1975. Nutrition in the United States, 1900 to 1974. *Cancer Research* 35:3246–3253.

Greenpeace. 2009. Fact sheet: The whale meat market in Japan. http://www .greenpeace.org/raw/content/international/press/reports/fact-sheet-the-whale -meat-mar.pdf

Hall, K., et al. 2009. The progressive increase of food waste in America and its environmental impact. *PLoS ONE* 4 (11):1–6.

Halliwell, B. 2007. Dietary polyphenols: Good, bad, or indifferent for your health? *Cardiovascular Research* 73:341–347.

Hanley, S. B. 1997. *Everyday Things in Premodern Japan.* Berkeley: University of California Press.

Harada, N. 1989. *Edo no ryōri shi: ryōribon to ryōri bunka* [江戶の料理史: 料理本と料理文化 *The History of Edo Cuisine: Cookbooks and Food Culture*]. Tokyo: Chūō kōronsha.

Harada, N. 2008. A peek at the meals of the people of Edo. *Food Culture* 12:2–6, 13:2–6. http://kiifc.kikkoman.co.jp/foodculture/pdf_13/e_008_012.pdf

Hayami, Y. 1988. *Japanese Agriculture under Siege: The Political Economy of Agricultural Policies.* New York: St. Martin's Press.

Hayami, Y., and V. W. Ruttan. 1970. Korean rice, Taiwan rice, and Japanese agricultural stagnation: An economic consequence of colonialism. *Quarterly Journal of Economics* 84:562–589.

Hayami, Y., and S. Yamada. 1970. Agricultural productivity at the beginning of industrialization. In *Agriculture and Economic Growth: Japan's Experience*, ed. K. Ohkawa, B. F. Johnston, and H. Kaneda, 105–129. Princeton, NJ: Princeton University Press.

Hayami, Y., and S. Yamada. 1991. *Agricultural Development of Japan: A Century's Perspective*. Tokyo: University of Tokyo Press.

Hayashi, K., S. Nishimura, and K. Yagi. 2006. Ammonia volatilization from the surface of a Japanese paddy filed during rice cultivation. *Soil Science and Plant Nutrition* 52:545–555.

Hayashi, R., and M. Amano. 2005. *Nihon no aji, shōyu no rekishi*. [Japan's Taste, History of Soy Sauce] Tokyo: Yoshikawa Kōbunkan.

Hayashi, Y. 2006. *Japan's Annual Southern Bluefin Tuna Catch Halved*. Tokyo: U.S. Department of Agriculture, Foreign Agricultural Service.

He, B., et al. 2009. Integrated biogeochemical modelling of nitrogen load from anthropogenic and natural sources in Japan. *Ecological Modelling* 220:2325–2334.

Hermanussen, M., et al. 2007. BMI in Japanese children since 1948: No evidence of a major rise in the prevalence of obesity in Japan. *Anthropologischer Anzeiger* 65:275–283.

Higeta shōyu. 2009. Corporate history. http://www.higeta.co.jp/en/company/enkaku.html

Hirai, Y., and H. Nishinokubi. 2004. By-catch and discards of marketable species for small-scale trawler in Ariake Sea. *Nippon Suisan Gakkai Shi* 70:738–744.

Hirohata, T., and S. Kono. 1997. Diet/nutrition and stomach cancer in Japan. *International Journal of Cancer* 10:34–36.

Hirono, Y., I. Watanabe, and K. Nonaka. 2009. Trends in water quality around an intensive tea-growing area in Shizuoka, Japan. *Soil Science and Plant Nutrition* 55:783–792.

Hoekstra, A. Y., ed. 2003. *Virtual Water Trade: Proceedings of the International Expert Meeting on Virtual Water Trade*. Delft: IHE.

Hoekstra, A. Y., and A. K. Chapagain. 2007. Water footprints of nations: Water use by people as a function of their consumption pattern. *Water Resources Management* 21:35–48.

Hoekstra, A. Y., and P. Q. Hung. 2005. Globalisation of water resources: international virtual water flows in relation to crop trade. *Global Environmental Change* 15:45–56.

Hori, T. 1992. *Maguro to Nihonjin*. [マグロと日本人 Tuna and the Japanese] Tokyo: Nihon Hōsō Shuppan Kyōkai.

Hori, T. 1996. Tuna and the Japanese: In *Search of a Sustainable Ecosystem*. Tokyo: Japan External Trade Organization.

Hosaka, T. A. 2011. Big tuna fetches record $396,000 in Tokyo. http://hosted2.ap.org/APDEFAULT/login/Article_2011-01-05-Japan%20Pricey%20Tuna/id-8aeb622d01dc48fe9d841667293809c3

Hoshiyama, Y., et al. 2004. A nested case-control study of stomach cancer in relation to green tea consumption in Japan. *British Journal of Cancer* 90:135–138.

Hosking, R. 1996. *A Dictionary of Japanese Food: Ingredients and Culture.* Boston: Tuttle Publishing.

Hui, Y. H., ed. 1993. *Dairy Science and Technology, Handbook 2: Product Manufacturing.* New York: VCH.

Inoue, M., et al. 2008. Green tea consumption and gastric cancer in Japanese: a pooled analysis of six cohort studies. *Gut* 58:1323–1332.

International Commission for the Conservation of Atlantic Tunas. 2009. *Statistical Bulletin.* http://www.iccat.es/Documents/SCRS/other/StatBull38pdf

International Institute of Agriculture. 1926. *International Yearbook of Agricultural Statistics 1925–26.* Rome: International Institute of Agriculture.

International Institute of Agriculture. 1937. *International Yearbook of Agricultural Statistics 1935–36 and 1936–37.* Rome: International Institute of Agriculture.

Institute of Cetacean Research. 2010. Japan's whale research programs. http://www.icrwhale.org/generalinfo.htm

International Rice Research Institute. 1979. *Nitrogen and Rice.* Los Baños, Philippines: IRRI.

International Rice Research Institute. 1987. *Efficiency of Nitrogen Fertilizers for Rice.* Los Baños, Philippines: International Rice Research Institute.

International Rice Research Institute. 2008. IRRI world rice statistics. Los Baños: International Rice Research Institute. http://www.irri.org/science/ricestat/data/may2008/WRS2008-AppendixTable05.pdf

International Rice Research Institute. 2009a. Japan. http://www.irri.org/science/cnyinfo/japan.asp

International Rice Research Institute. 2009b. Rice calorie supply as percentage of total calorie supply, by country and geographical region, 1961–2005. http://beta.irri.org/solutions/images/stories/wrs/wrs_jul30_2009_table17_consumption_USDA.xls

International Sugar Organization. 2009. *Sugar Year Book 2008.* http://www.isosugar.org/Publications/PFD%20files/SYB%20Introduction.pdf

Isanga, J., and G. Zhang. 2008. Soybean bioactive components and their implications to health—A review. *Food Reviews International* 24:252–276.

Ishida, M. 2009. Whaling library. http://luna.pos.to/whale

Ishige, N. 2000. Japan. In *The Cambridge World History of Food,* ed. K. F. Kiple and K. C. Ornelas, 1175–1183. Cambridge: Cambridge University Press.

Ishige, N. 2001. *The History and Culture of Japanese Food.* London: Kegan Paul.

Ishihara, A., and J. Yoshii. 2003. A survey of the commercial trade in whale meat products in Japan. Tokyo: TRAFFIC East Asia–Japan. http://www.traffic.org/mammals

Issenberg, S. 2007. *The Sushi Economy.* New York: Gotham Books.

Ito, H. 2008. Japan's use of flour began with noodles. *Food Culture* 16:1–4. http://kiifc.kikkoman.co.jp/foodculture/pdf_16/e_001_004.pdf

Jannetta, A. B. 1992. Famine mortality in nineteenth-century Japan: The evidence from a temple death register. *Population Studies* 46:427–443.

Japan Fertilizer and Ammonia Producers Association. 2010. JFA. http://www.jaf .gr.jp/english/english.htm

Japan Sake Brewers Association. 2010. Types of sake. http://www.japansake .or.jp/sake/english/types_sake.html

Japan Soft Drink Association. 2009. ソフトドリンク品目別生産量の推移 [Changes in soft drink production by items]. http://www.j-sda.or.jp/about-jsda/sd-statistics/ stati02.html

Japan for Sustainability. 2009. Survey shows growing awareness of Japan's food self-sufficiency rate. http://www.japanfs.org/en/pages/029028.html

Kako, T. 2004. Trend of rice consumption in Japan. http://worldfood.apionet .or.jp/kankoku/Japan/5Kako.ppt

Kalland, A., and B. Moeran. 1992. *Japanese Whaling: End of an Era?* London: Curzon Press.

Kamekura, J., M. Watanabe, and H. Bosker. 1989. *Ekiben: The Art of the Japanese Lunchbox.* San Francisco: Chronicle Books.

Kanade, A. N., M. K. Gokhale, and S. Rao. 2001. Energy costs of standard activities among Indian adults. *European Journal of Clinical Nutrition* 55: 708–713.

Kaneda, H. 1970. Long-term changes in food consumption patterns in Japan. In *Agriculture and Economic Growth: Japan's Experience*, ed. K. Ohkawa, B. F. Johnston, and H. Kaneda, 398–429. Princeton, NJ: Princeton University Press.

Katanoda, K., and Y. Matsumura. 2002. National Nutrition Survey in Japan—Its methodological transition and current findings. *Journal of Nutritional Science and Vitaminology* 48:423–432.

Katanoda, K., et al. 2005. Is the national nutrition survey in Japan representative of the entire Japanese population? *Nutrition (Burbank, Los Angeles County, Calif.)* 21:964–966.

Kawamura, Y., and M. R. Kare, eds. 1987. *Umami, a Basic Taste: Physiology, Biochemistry, Nutrition, Food Science.* New York: Marcel Dekker.

Kazuko, E. 2001. *Japanese Food and Cooking: A Timeless Cuisine.* London: Lorenz Books.

Keferl, M. 2008. Placenta 10000 jelly drink is FOSHU for beauty. http://www .japantrends.com/placenta-10000-jelly-drink-is-foshu-for-beauty

Kelleher, K. 2004. *Discards in the World's Marine Fisheries: An Update.* Rome: Food and Agriculture Organization.

Keys, A., ed. 1970. *Coronary Heart Disease in Seven Countries.* New York: American Heart Association.

KFC Japan. 2010. ケンタッキーフライドチキン [Kentucky Fried Chicken]. http:// www.kfc.co.jp

Kikkoman. 2010. Corporate profile: History. http://www.kikkoman.com/corporateprofile/history/index.shtml

Kikuchi, N., et al. 2006. No association between green tea and prostate cancer risk in Japanese men: the Ohsaki Cohort Study. *British Journal of Cancer* 95:371–373.

Kimura, A. H., and M. Nishiyama. 2008. The *chisan-chisho* movement: Japanese local food movement and its challenges. *Agriculture and Human Values* 25:49–64.

Kimuraya. 2010. *Kimuraya* 木村屋 http://www.ginzakimuraya.jp.

King, F. H. 1911. *Farmers of Forty Centuries, or, Permanent Agriculture in China, Korea and Japan*. Madison, WI: F. H. King.

Kinsella, K. G. 1992. Changes in life expectancy 1900–1990. *American Journal of Clinical Nutrition* 55:1196S–1202S.

Kit Kat. 2009. Breaktown. http://www.breaktown.com/omiyage

Kokubo, Y., et al. 2007. Association of dietary intake of soy, beans, and isoflavones with risk of cerebral and myocardial infarctions in Japanese populations—The Japan Public Health Center-Based (JPHC) Study Cohort I. *Circulation* 116:2553–2562.

Kondo, H. 1984. *Sake: A Drinker's Guide*. Tokyo: Kōdansha.

Kozlov, A. I., et al. 1998. Gene geography of primary hypolactasia in populations of the Old World. *Genetika* 34:551–561.

Kumazawa, K. 2002. Nitrogen fertilization and nitrate pollution in groundwater in Japan: Present status and measures for sustainable agriculture. *Nutrient Cycling in Agroecosystems* 63:129–137.

Kurihara, H. 2006. *Harumi's Japanese Cooking: More Than 75 Authentic and Contemporary Recipes from Japan's Most Popular Cooking Expert*. New York: HP Trade.

Kuriyama, S., et al. 2006. Green tea consumption and mortality due to cardiovascular disease, cancer, and all causes in Japan: the Ohsaki study. *Journal of the American Medical Association* 296:1255–1265.

Kwok, R. H. M. 1968. Chinese-restaurant syndrome. *New England Journal of Medicine* 278:796.

Kyoto Kokuritsu Hakubutsukan. 2002. *Nihonjin to cha*. [日本人と茶 Japanese and Tea:] Kyoto: KKH.

Lee, W. T. K. 2002. Nutrition transition in China—a challenge in the new millennium. *Nutrition and Dietetics* 59:74.

Lichtenstein, A. H., and L. Van Horn. 1998. Very low fat diets. *Circulation* 98:935–939.

Lipoeto, N. I., et al. 2004. Nutrition transition in West Sumatra, Indonesia. *Asia Pacific Journal of Clinical Nutrition* 13:312–316.

Longworth, J. W. 1983. *Beef in Japan: Politics, Production, Marketing and Trade*. St. Lucia: University of Queensland.

Lowenstein, J. H., G. Amato, and S. Kolokotronis. 2009. The real *maccoyii*: Identifying tuna sushi with DNA barcodes—Contrasting characteristic attributes and genetic distances. *PLoS ONE* 4 (11):1–14.

MacKenzie, B. R., H. Mosegaard, and A. A. Rosenberg. 2009. Impending collapse of bluefin tuna in the northeast Atlantic and Mediterranean. *Conservation Letters* 2:25–34.

Mak, J., L. Carlile, and S. Dai. 2004. *Impact of Population Aging on Japanese International Travel to 2025.* Honolulu, HI: East West Center. http://www.eastwestcenter.org/fileadmin/stored/pdfs/ECONwp073.pdf.

Mashimo, T. 2008. To what level could Japan's food self-sufficiency recover? *Japan Resources* no. 147. http://www.nishoren.org/en/?p=287 (accessed in March 2009)

Masia, R., et al. 1999. High prevalence of cardiovascular risk factors in Gerona, Spain, a province with low myocardial infarction incidence. *Journal of Epidemiology and Community Health* 52:707–715.

Masuma, S., et al. 2008. Status of bluefin tuna farming, broodstock management, breeding and fingerling production in Japan. *Reviews in Fisheries Science* 16:385–390.

Matsumoto, H. 2006. The world's thriving sushi business. *Food Culture* 13:1–5. http://kiifc.kikkoman.co.jp/foodculture/pd_13/e_008_012.pdf

Matsumoto, H. 2008. The internalization of sushi. *Food Culture* 15:1–5. http://kiifc.kikkoman.co.jp/foodculture/pdf_15/e_002_006.pdf

Matsushita, Y., et al. 2009. Taste preferences and body weight change in Japanese adults: The JPHC Study. *International Journal of Obesity* 33:1191–1197.

Matsuzaka, M., et al. 2007. The decreasing burden of gastric cancer in Japan. *Tohoku Journal of Experimental Medicine* 212:207–219.

McCay, C. M., M. F. Crowell, and L. A. Maynard. 1935. The effect of retarded growth upon the length of the life-span and ultimate body size. *Journal of Nutrition* 10:63–79.

McDonald's Japan. 2010. 日本マクドナルド [*Nihon Makudonarudo*]. http://www.mcdonalds.co.jp

McHugh, D. J. 2003. *A Guide to the Seaweed Industry.* Rome: FAO.

Menotti, A., et al. 1999. Food intake patterns and 25-year mortality from coronary heart disease: Cross-cultural correlations in the Seven Countries Study. *European Journal of Epidemiology* 15:507–515.

Messina, M., C. Nagata, and A. H. Wu. 2006. Estimated Asian adult soy protein and isoflavone intakes. *Nutrition and Cancer* 55:1–12.

Ministry of Agriculture, Forestry, and Fisheries. 2006. Fisheries of Japan–2006/2007. http://www.maff.go.jp/e/pdf/fy2006.pdf.

Ministry of Agriculture, Forestry, and Fisheries. 2007. Proposal for Japanese Restaurant Recommendation Program (Draft). http://www.mff.go.jp/e/soushoku/sanki/easia/e_sesaku/japanese_food/pdf/proposal_e.pdf.

Ministry of Agriculture, Forestry, and Fisheries. 2008a. *Annual Report on Food, Agriculture and Rural Areas in Japan FY 2008*. http://www.maff.go.jp/e/annual_report/2008/index.html.

Ministry of Agriculture, Forestry, and Fisheries. 2008b. Fisheries of Japan 2008/2009: Fisheries policy outline for FY2009 (White Paper on Fisheries). http://www.jfa.maff.go.jp/e/annual_report/2008/index.html.

Ministry of Agriculture, Forestry, and Fisheries. 2010. *The 85th Statistical Yearbook of Ministry of Agriculture, Forestry and Fisheries (2009~2010)*. Tokyo: Ministry of Agriculture, Forestry and Fisheries. http://www.maff.go.jp/e/tokei/kikaku/nenji_e/85nnji/index.html.

Ministry of Environment. 2006. *Annual Report on the Environment in Japan 2006*. http://www.env.go.jp/en/wpaper/2006/fulltext.pdf.

Ministry of Environment. 2008. *Annual Report on the Environment and the Sound Material-Cycle Society in Japan 2008*. Tokyo: Ministry of Environment. http://www.env.go.jp/en/wpaper/2008/index.html.

Ministry of Health, Labour, and Welfare. 2004. *Dietary Reference Intakes for Japanese* (2005). Tokyo: Ministry of Health, Labour, and Welfare. http://www.nih.go.jp/eiken/english/research/pdf/dris2005_eng.pdf.

Ministry of Health, Labour, and Welfare. 2009. *Outline for the Results of the National Health and Nutrition Survey Japan, 2006*. Tokyo: Ministry of Health, Labour, and Welfare. http://www.nih.go.jp/eiken/english/research/pdf/nhns2006_outline.pdf.

Ministry of Health and Welfare. 1995. Japan's average life expectancy remains highest in world. *Information Bulletin*, no. 19.

Minami, K. 2005. N cycle, N flow trends in Japan, and strategies for reducing N2O emissions and NO3 pollution. *Pedosphere* 15:164–172.

Mishima, S. 2001. Recent trend of nitrogen flow associated with agricultural production in Japan. *Soil Science and Plant Nutrition* 45:881–889.

Mishima, S., A. Endo, and K. Kohyama. 2009. Recent trend in residual nitrogen on national and regional scales in Japan and its relation with groundwater quality. *Nutrient Cycling in Agroecosystems* 83:1–11.

Mishima, S., N. Matsumoto, and K. Oda. 1999. Nitrogen flow associated with agricultural practices and environmental risk in Japan. *Soil Science and Plant Nutrition* 45:881–889.

Mishima, S., S. Taniguchi, and M. Komada. 2006. Recent trends in nitrogen and phosphate use and balance on Japanese farmland. *Soil Science and Plant Nutrition* 52:556–563.

Mitsubishi Economic Research Bureau. 1936. *Japanese Trade and Industry: Present and Future*. London: Macmillan.

Miura, I. 2009. Japanese tofu industry. http://www.midwestshippers.com/conferencePresentations/JapaneseTofuMarket.pdf.

Miyabe, N. 2003. Description of the Japanese longline fishery and its fishery statistics in the Mediterranean Sea during the recent years. *Collective Volume of Scientific Papers ICCAT* 55:131–137.

Miyake, M. P., N. Miyabe, and H. Nakano. 2004. *Historical Trends of Tuna Catches in the World*. Rome: Food and Agriculture Organization.

Miyashita, A. 2000. *Katsuobushi*. [鰹節 Katsuobushi] Tokyo: Hōsei Daigaku Shuppankyōku.

Miyashita, A. 2004. *Nori no rekishi* [海苔の歴史 *History of nori*]. Tokyo: Kaiji shōin.

Molden, D., ed. 2007. *Water for Food Water for Life*. London: Earthscan.

Mori, K. 1950. *Shiitake*. [椎茸 Shiitake] Tokyo: Yūtosha.

Morishima, M., ed. 1990. *Suiden nōgyō no genjō to yosoku* [水田農業の現状と予測 Present conditions of paddy field agriculture. Tokyo: Fumin kyōkai.

Morimoto, M. 2007. *Morimoto: The New Art of Japanese Cooking*. New York: Doris Kindersley.

Morris-Suzuki, T. 1994. *The Technological Transformation of Japan: From the Seventeenth to the Twenty-First Century*. Cambridge: Cambridge University Press.

Mosk, C. 1978. Fecundity, infanticide, and food consumption in Japan. *Explorations in Economic History* 15:269–289.

Mosk, C., and S. Pak. 1978. *Food Consumption, Physical Characteristics, and Population Growth in Japan, 1874–1940*. Berkeley: Department of Economics, University of California at Berkeley.

Murano, K., et al. 1995. Gridded ammonia emission fluxes in Japan. *Water, Air, and Soil Pollution* 85:1915–1920.

Murata, M. 2000. Secular trends in growth and changes in eating patterns of Japanese children. *American Journal of Clinical Nutrition* 72:1379S–1383S.

Muto, F., et al. 2009. Pacific bluefin tuna fisheries in Japan and adjacent areas before the mid-20th century. http://www.iccat.int/Documents/Meetings/Docs/BFT_SYMP/pdf/BFT_SYMP_032.pdf

MyVoice. 2007. Almost four in five Japanese eat rice daily. *What Japan Thinks*. http://whatjapanthinks.com/2007/02/05/almost-four-in-five-japanese-eat-rice-daily

Naganuma, T., et al. 2009. Green tea consumption and hematologic malignancies in Japan. *American Journal of Epidemiology* 170:730–738.

Nagata, C., et al. 2001. Soy product intake and hot flashes in Japanese women: Results from a community-based prospective study. *American Journal of Epidemiology* 153:790–793.

Nagata, C., et al. 2002. A prospective cohort study of soy product intake and stomach cancer death. *British Journal of Cancer* 87:31–36.

Nagata, Y., et al. 2007. Dietary isoflavones may protect against prostate cancer in Japanese men. *Journal of Nutrition* 137:1974–1979.

Nagura, J., et al. 2009. Fruit, vegetable and bean intake and mortality from cardiovascular disease among Japanese men and women: The JACC study. *British Journal of Nutrition* 102:285–292.

Nakamura, E. G. 2000. Physicians and famine in Japan: Takano Choei in the 1830s. *Social History of Medicine* 13:429–445.

Nakamura, J. 1966. *Agricultural Production and the Economic Development of Japan*. Princeton, NJ: Princeton University Press.

Nakamura, K., et al. 2008. Fruit and vegetable intake and mortality from cardiovascular disease are inversely associated in Japanese women but not in men. *Journal of Nutrition* 138:1129–1134.

Nakata, T. 2003. A Study on the volume and transportation distance as to food imports ("food mileage") and its influence on the environment. *Journal of Agricultural Policy Research* 5:45–59.

Nakayama, S. 1967. Long-term changes in food consumption in Japan. *Developing Economies* 7:220–232.

Nasu, S. 1927. *The Problem of Population and Food Supply in Japan*. Honolulu, HI: Institute of Pacific Relations.

National Cancer Center. 2009. Cancer statistics in Japan. http://ganjoho.ncc .go.jp/public/statistics/backnumber/1isaao000000068m-att/fig11.pdf

National Institutes of Health. 2009. *Morbidity and Mortality: 2009 Chart Book on Cardiovascular, Lung and Blood Diseases*. Bethesda, MD: National Institutes of Health.

Nippon Research Center. 2006. Opinion poll on scientific whaling. Tokyo: Greenpeace Japan. http://www.greenpeace.org/raw/content/international/press/ reports/whaling-poll-japan.pdf.

Nishio, K., et al. 2007. Consumption of soy foods and the risk of breast cancer: Findings from the Japan Collaborative Cohort (JACC) Study. *Cancer Causes and Control* 18:801–808.

Nishiyama, M. 1997. *Edo Culture: Daily Life and Diversions in Urban Japan, 1600–1868*. Honolulu: University of Hawaii Press.

Nissin Foods. 2010. About the inventor. http://www.nissinfoods.com/company/ about.php.

Niu, K., et al. 2009. Green tea consumption is associated with depressive symptoms in the elderly. *American Journal of Clinical Nutrition* 90:1615–1622.

Nobu. 2009. New Year's Eve Thursday, December 31, 2009. http://www .myriadrestaurantgroup.com/nobu/index.html

National Obesity Observatory. 2009. International Comparisons of Adult Obesity Prevalence. http://www.noo.org.uk/NOO_about_obesity/international

Norinchukin Bank. 2008. 海外旅行から帰ってきたら食べたくなる物ランキング [Ranking of meals to eat after returning from a trip abroad]. http://ranking.goo .ne.jp/ranking/013/gethome_food

Oba, S., et al. 2009. Diet based on the Japanese food guide spinning top and subsequent mortality among men and women in a general Japanese population. *Journal of the American Dietetic Association* 109:1540–1547.

Obara, K. 2009. *2009 Outlook for Fluid Milk, NFDM, Butter and Cheese*. Tokyo: USDA Foreign Agricultural Service.

Obara, K., J. Dyck, and J. Stout. 2005. *Dairy Policies in Japan*. Washington, DC: USDA.

Ocké, M.C., et al. 2009. Energy intake and sources of energy intake in the European Prospective Investigation into Cancer and Nutrition. *European Journal of Clinical Nutrition* 63:S3–D15.

Ogura, T. 1980. *Can Japanese Agriculture Survive? A Historical and Comparative Approach*. Tokyo: Agricultural Policy Research Center.

Oh, K., et al. 2006. Environmental problems from tea cultivation in Japan and a control measure using calcium cyanamide. *Pedosphere* 16:770–777.

Ohki, S. 2009. *Tea Culture of Japan*. New Haven, CT: Yale University Art Gallery.

Ohnishi, M. 1995. *Mrs. Ohnishi's Whale Cuisine*. Tokyo: Kōdansha International.

Ohnuki-Tierney, E. 1993. *Rice as Self: Japanese Identities through Time*. Princeton, NJ: Princeton University Press.

Okamoto, H. 2004. Search for the Japanese tuna fishing data before and just after World War II. *Bulletin of Fisheries Research Agency* 13:15–34.

Okamoto, M. 2006. River resources allocation and participatory irrigation management in Japan today. *Journal of Developments in Sustainable Agriculture* 1:41–43.

Ōkawa, K., M. Ito, and T. Noda. 1957. *The Growth Rate of the Japanese Economy since 1878*. Tokyo: Kinokuniya.

Ōkawa, K., B. F. Johnston, and H. Kaneda, eds. 1970. *Agriculture and Economic Growth: Japan's Experience*. Princeton, NJ: Princeton University Press.

Ōkawa, K., M. Shinohara, and M. Umemura eds. 1987–88. *Chōki keizai tōkei* [*Estimates of Long-Term Economic Statistics*] Tokyo: Tōyō keizai shinpōsha.

Oki, T., et al. 2003. Virtual water trade to Japan and in the world. In: A.Y. Hoekstra, ed., *Virtual Water Trade: Proceedings of the International Expert Meeting on Virtual Water Trade*, Delft: IHE, pp. 221–235.

Ōmameuda, M. 2007. *Okome to shoku no kindaishi*. [お米と食の近代史 Modern History of Rice and Foods] Tokyo: Yoshikawa-Kōbunkan.

Ooms, H. 1996. *Tokugawa Village Practice: Class, Status, Power, Law*. Berkeley: University of California Press.

Organization for Economic Cooperation and Development. 2009. *OECD in Figures 2009*. Paris: Organization for Economic Cooperation and Development.

Pauly, D. 2009. Beyond duplicity and ignorance in global fisheries. *Scientia Marina* 73:215–224.

Pauly, D., et al. 1998. Fishing down marine food webs. *Science* 279:860–863.

Pauly, D., et al. 2000. Fishing down aquatic food webs. *American Scientist* 88:46–51.

Perry, M. C. 1856. *Narrative of the Expedition of an American Squadron to the China Seas and Japan, Performed in the Years 1852, 1853, and 1854 under the*

Command of Commodore M.C. Perry, United States Navy, by Order of the Government of the United States. Washington, DC: U.S. Congress.

Phelan, J. P., and M. R. Rose. 2005. Why dietary restriction substantially increases longevity in animal models but won't in humans. *Ageing Research Reviews* 4:339–350.

Phelan, J. P., and M. R. Rose. 2006. Caloric restriction increases longevity substantially only when the reaction norm is steep. *Biogerontology* 7:161–164.

Polacheck, T., and C. Davies. 2008. *Considerations of Implications of Large Unreported Catches of Southern Bluefin Tuna for Assessments of Tropical Tunas, and the Need for Independent Verification of Catch and Effort Statistics.* http:// www.iotc.org/files/proceedings/2008/wptt/IOTC-2008-WPTT-INF01.pdf.

Popkin, B. M. 2003. Nutrition transition: Worldwide diet change. In: *Gale Encyclopedia of Food and Culture.* http://www.answers.com/topic/nutrition -transition-worldwide-diet-change.

Portinari, F., et al. 1989. Il manifesto dello slow-food. http://editore.slowfood.it/ editore/riviste/slowfood/IT/19/articoli/slowfood19_05.pdf.

Przybylowicz, P., and J. Donoghue. 1988. *Shiitake Growers Handbook: The Art and Science of Mushroom Cultivation.* Dubuque, IA: Kendall/Hunt.

Raiten, D. J., J. M. Talbot, and K. D. Fisher, eds. 1995. *Analysis of Adverse Reactions to Monosodium Glutamate (MSG).* Bethesda, MD: American Society for Experimental Biology.

Ralston, K., C. Newman, A. Clauson, J. Guthrie, and J. Buzby. 2008. *The National School Lunch Program: Background, Trends, and Issues.* Washington, DC: USDA. http://www.ers.usda.gov/publications/err61/err61.pdf.

Rath, E. C. 2010. *Food and Fantasy in Early Modern Japan.* Berkeley: University of California Press.

Rath, E. C., and S. Assmann, eds. 2010. *Japanese Foodways, Past and Present.* Urbana: University of Illinois Press.

Renaud, S., and M. de Lorgeril. 1992. Wine, alcohol, platelets, and the French paradox for coronary heart disease. *Lancet* 339:1523–1526.

Richie, D. 1985. *A Taste of Japan.* Tokyo: Kōdansha International.

Sacks, F. M., et al. 2006. Soy protein, isoflavones, and cardiovascular health. *Circulation* 113:1034–1044.

Saga, J. 1987. *Memories of Silk and Straw: A Self-Portrait of Small-Town Japan.* Tokyo: Kōdansha International.

Sakata, S., and M. Moriyama. 1990. Japanese dietary intake of salt and protein. *Tohoku Journal of Experimental Medicine* 162:293–302.

Salt Industry Center of Japan. 2009. Changes in quantity of salt intake. http:// www.shiojigyo.com/english/data/changes.html

Sanfeliu, C., et al. 2003. Neurotoxicity of organomercurial compounds. *Neurotoxicity Research* 5:283–305.

Sano, S., J. Yanai, and T. Kosaki. 2004. Evaluation of soil nitrogen status in Japanese agricultural lands with reference to land use and soil types. *Soil Science and Plant Nutrition* 50:501–510.

Sarhage, D., and J. Lundbeck. 1992. *A History of Fishing*. Berlin: Springer-Verlag.

Sasamoto, T., et al. 2006. Estimation of 1999–2004 dietary daily intake of PCDDs, PCDFs and dioxin-like PCBs by a total diet study in metropolitan Tokyo, Japan. *Chemosphere* 64:634–641.

Sato, H. 2001. The current state of paddy agriculture in Japan. *Irrigation and Drainage* 50:91–99.

Sauvaget, C., et al. 2003a. Vegetable and fruit intake and stroke mortality in the Hiroshima/Nagasaki Life Span Study. *Stroke* 34:2355–2360.

Sauvaget, C., et al. 2003b. Intake of animal products and stroke mortality in the Hiroshima/Nagasaki Life Span Study. *International Journal of Epidemiology* 32:543–545.

Sekikawa, A., et al. 2003. A "natural experiment" in cardiovascular epidemiology in the early 21st century. *Heart (British Cardiac Society)* 89:255–257.

Seven Countries Study. 2009. Seven Countries Study: Japan. http://www.epi.umn.edu/research/7countries/japan.shtm.

Shetty, P. S. 2002. Nutrition transition in India. *Public Health Nutrition* 5 (1A):175–182.

Shiba, T. 1986. *Kujira to Nihonjin*. [[鯨と日本人 Whales and the Japanese]] Tokyo: Yōsensha.

Shimazu, T., et al. 2007. Dietary patterns and cardiovascular disease mortality in Japan: A prospective cohort study. *International Journal of Epidemiology* 36:600–609.

Shinohara, M. 1967. *Kojin shōhi shishutsu [Personal consumption expenditure] Chōki keizai tōkei [Long-term economic statistics]*, vol. 6. Tokyo: Keizai Shinpōsha.

Sho, H. 2001. History and characteristics of Okinawan longevity food. *Asia Pacific Journal of Clinical Nutrition* 10:159–164.

Shurtleff, W., and A. Aoyagi. 1975. *The Book of Tofu*. New York: Ballantine Books.

Shurtleff, W., and A. Aoyagi. 2007. *History of Soybeans and Soyfoods: 1100 B.C. to the 1980s*. Lafayette, CA: Soyinfo Center.

Simmonds, M. P., et al. 2002. Human health significance of organochlorine and mercury contaminants in Japanese whale meat. *Journal of Toxicology and Environmental Health* 65:1211–1235.

Simoons, F. J. 1978. The geographic hypothesis and lactose malabsorption: A weighing of evidence. *American Journal of Digestive Diseases* 23:963–980.

Smil, V. 1999. China's great famine: Forty years later. *British Medical Journal* 7225:1619–1621.

Smil, V. 2000. *Feeding the World*. Cambridge, MA: MIT Press.

Smil, V. 2001. *Agricultural Harvests, Total Crop Phytomass Production and Rising Yields in Six Nations During the 20th Century*. Unpublished report prepared for INSEAD, Paris.

Smil, V. 2002. Eating meat: Evolution, patterns, and consequences. *Population and Development Review* 28:599–639.

Smil, V. 2004. *China's Past, China's Future*. London: RoutledgeCurzon.

Smil, V. 2005. Feeding the world: How much more rice do we need? In *Rice Is Life: Scientific Perspectives for the 21st Century. Proceedings of the World Rice Research Conference Held in Tokyo and Tsukuba, Japan, 4–7 November 2004*, ed. K. Toriyama, K. L. Heong, and B. Hardy. Los Baños: International Rice Research Institute, 21–23.

Smil, V. 2008. *Energy in Nature and Society*. Cambridge, MA: MIT Press.

Smil, V. 2009. Two decades later: Nikkei and lessons from the fall. *American*, December 29, 2009. http://www.american.com/archive/2009/december-2009/two-decades-later-nikkei-and-lessons-from-the-fall.

Sohal, R. S., and R. Weindruch. 1996. Oxidative stress, caloric restriction, and aging. *Science* 273:59–63.

Sone, T., et al. 2008. Sense of life worth living (*ikigai*) and mortality in Japan: Ohsaki Study. *Psychosomatic Medicine* 70:709–715.

Sonu, S. C. 2006. *Albacore Fisheries, Trade, and Market of Japan, 2005*. Long Beach, CA: U.S. Department of Commerce. http://swr.nmfs.noaa.gov/fmd/sunee/tm-43.pdf.

Sonu, S. C. 2007. *Bigeye Tuna Fisheries, Trade, and Market of Japan*. Long Beach, CA: U.S. Department of Commerce. http://swr.nmfs.noaa.gov/fmd/sunee/BigeyeTuna2007.pdf.

Sonu, S. C. 2008. *Bluefin Tuna Supply, Demand and Market of Japan*. Long Beach, CA: U.S. Department of Commerce. http://swr.nmfs.noaa.gov/fmd/sunee/bluefin.pdf.

Speakman, J. R., and C. Hambly. 2007. Starving for life: What animal studies can and cannot tell us about the use of caloric restriction to prolong human lifespan. *Journal of Nutrition* 137:1078–1086.

Starbuck, A. 1989. *History of the American Whale Fishery*. Secaucus, NJ: Castle.

Statistics Bureau. 2011a. *Historical Statistics of Japan*. Tokyo: Statistics Bureau. http://www.stat.go.jp/english/data/chouki/index.htm.

Statistics Bureau. 2011b. *Japan Statistical Yearbook 2011*. Tokyo: Statistics Bureau. http://www.stat.go.jp/english/data/nenkan/index.htm.

Stevenson, D. D. 2000. Monosodium glutamate and asthma. *Journal of Nutrition* 130:1067S–1073S.

Strazzullo, P., et al. 2009. Salt intake, stroke, and cardiovascular disease: Meta-analysis of prospective studies. *British Medical Journal* 339:b4567.

Suarez, F. L., and D. A. Savaiano. 1997. Diet, genetics, and lactose intolerance. *Food Technology* 51:74–76.

Sugawara, Y., et al. 2009. Fish consumption and the risk of colorectal cancer: The Ohsaki cohort study. *British Journal of Cancer* 101:849–854.

Sun, Y. C., et al. 2007. Lifestyle and overweight among Japanese adolescents: Toyama birth cohort study. *Journal of Epidemiology* 19:303–310.

Swartz, W. K. 2000. *Global Maps of the Growth of Japanese Marine Fisheries and Fish Consumption*. Vancouver, BC: University of British Columbia.

Syokuryo. 2010. Food Action Nippon. http://syokuryo.jp/index.html.

Takachi, R., et al. 2008. Fruit and vegetable intake and risk of total cancer and cardiovascular disease. *American Journal of Epidemiology* 167:59–70.

Takahashi, E. 1984. Secular trend in milk consumption and growth in Japan. *Human Biology* 56:427–437.

Tamura, T. 1966. *Marine Aquaculture*. Washington, DC: U.S. Department of Commerce.

Tanaka, Y. 1998. The cyclical sensibility of Edo-period Japan. *Japan Echo* 25 (2):12–16.

Tanaka, Y., and Y. Sato. 2005. Farmers managed irrigation districts in Japan: Assessing how fairness may contribute to sustainability. *Agricultural Water Management* 77:196–209.

Tian, Y., H. Kidokoro, and T. Watanabe. 2006. Long-term changes in the fish community structure from the Tsushima warm current region of the Japan/East Sea with an emphasis on the impacts of fishing and climate regime shift over the last four decades. *Progress in Oceanography* 68:217–237.

Tokui, N., et al. 2005. Dietary habits and stomach cancer risk in the JACC study. *Journal of Epidemiology* 15:S98–S108.

Toriyama, K. 2002. Estimation of fertilizer nitrogen requirement for average rice yield in Japanese paddy fields. *Soil Science and Plant Nutrition* 48:293–300.

Toshima, H., Y. Koga, and H. Blackburn, eds. 1994. *Lessons for Science from the Seven Countries Study*. Tokyo: Springer.

Truong-Minh, P., et al. 2009. Fish intake and the risk of fatal prostate cancer: Findings from a cohort study in Japan. *Public Health Nutrition* 12:609–613.

Tsubaki, T., and H. Takahashi, eds. 1986. *Recent Advances in Minamata Disease Studies: Methylmercury Poisoning in Minamata and Niigata, Japan*. Tokyo: Kodansha.

Tsubono, Y., et al. 1997. Dietary differences with green tea intake among middle-aged Japanese men and women. *Preventive Medicine* 26:704–710.

Tsuji, S. 1980. *Japanese Cooking: A Simple Art*. Tokyo: Kodansha International.

Tsukuba, H. 1986. *Beishoku, nikushoku no bunmei*. [Civilizations of Rice Consumption and Meat Consumption] Tokyo: Nihon Hōsō Shuppankai.

Uchida, E. 1989. *Edomae no sushi*. [江戸前の鮨 Edomae Sushi] Tokyo: Shōbunsha.

Udesky, J. 1988. *The Book of Soba*. Tokyo: Kōdansha.

Umemura, M., N. Takamatsu, and S. Itoh. 1983. *Chiiki Keizai Tōkei* (Regional Economic Statistics) In *Chōki Keizai Tōkei* (Long-Term Economic Statistics of Japan), Volume 13. Tokyo: Tōyō Keizai.

Umesawa, M., et al. 2009. Dietary calcium intake and risks of stroke, its subtypes, and coronary heart disease in Japanese. *Stroke* 39:2449–2456.

United Nations 2009. *World Population Prospects: The 2008 Revision*. http://esa.un.org/unpp

Uppal, J. N. 1984. *Bengal Famine of 1943: A Man-Made Tragedy*. Delhi: Atma Ram.

U.S. Bureau of the Census. 1975. *Historical Statistics of the United States: Colonial*. Washington, DC: US Bureau of the Census.

U.S. Department of Agriculture. 2008. *Agricultural Statistics 2008*. Washington, DC: USDA.Van der Meer, C. L. J., and S. Yamada. 1990. *Japanese Agriculture: A Comparative Economic Analysis*. Lodon: Routledge.

Varley, P., and I. Kumakura. 1989. *Tea in Japan: Essays on the History of chanoyu*. Honolulu: University of Hawaii Press.

Wakimoto, K. 2004. Utilization advantages of controlled release nitrogen fertilizer on paddy rice cultivation. *Japan Agricultural Research Quarterly* 38:15–20.

Waste and Resources Action Programme. 2008. *The Food We Waste*. http://www.wrap.org.uk/downloads/The_Food_We_Waste_v2__2_.cefd1ae9.5635.pdf.

Watanabe, I., et al. 2009. Green tea and death from pneumonia in Japan: The Ohsaki cohort study. *American Journal of Clinical Nutrition* 90:672–679.

Watanabe, T. 1989. *Nihonjin to inasaku bunka* (The Japanese and rice culture). *Nikkan Āgama* 103:81–91.

Watanabe, T., and A. Kishi. 1984. *The Book of Soybeans: Nature's Miracle Protein*. Tokyo: Kōdansha.

Watanabe, Y., and N. Suzuki. 2006. Is Japan's milk consumption saturated? *Journal of Faculty of Agriculture. Kyushu University* 51:165–171.

Watanabe, Z. 2004. The flavor of Edo spans the globe. *Food Culture* 7:1–6. http://kiifc.kikkoman.co.jp/foodculture/pdf_07/e_009_014.pdf.

Watanabe, Z. 2008. The meat-eating culture of Japan at the beginning of Westernization. *Food Culture* 9:2–8. http://kiifc.kikkoman.co.jp/foodculture/pdf_09/e_002_008.pdf.

Watson, R., and D. Pauly. 2001. Systematic distortions in world fisheries catch trends. *Nature* 414:534–536.

Weigold, A. 1999. Famine management: The Bengal famine (1942–1944) revisited. *South Asia* 33:63–77.

Weindruch, R., and R. L. Walford. 1988. *The Retardation of Aging and Disease by Dietary Restriction*. Springfield, IL: Charles C. Thomas.

Weng, X., and B. Caballero. 2007. *Obesity and Its Related Diseases in China: The Impact of the Nutrition Transition in Urban and Rural Adults.* Youngstown, NY: Cambria Press.

Whaling Library. 2010. Whaling statistics. http://luna.pos.to/whale/sta.html.

Wilcox, B. J., et al. 2007. Caloric restriction, the traditional Okinawan diet, and healthy aging. *Annals of the New York Academy of Sciences* 1114:434–455.

Wilcox, D. C., et al. 2006. Caloric restriction and human longevity: what can we learn from the Okinawans? *Biogerontology* 7:173–177.

World Database of Happiness. 2009. World database of happiness. http://worlddatabaseofhappiness.eur.nl/statnat/statnat_fp.htm

World Health Organization. 2009. WHO Oral Health Country/Area Profile Programme: Japan. Geneva: World Health Organization. http://www.whocollab.od.mah.se/wpro/japan/japan.html.

World Instant Noodles Association. 2010. History. http://instantnoodles.org/noodles/history.html.

World Meteorological Organization. 2010. *WMO Greenhouse Gas Bulletin.* Geneva: World Meteorological Organization. http://www.wmo.int/pages/prog/arep/gaw/ghg/documents/GHG_bull_6en.pdf.

WTO (World Trade Organization). 2011. *International Trade Statistics 2011.* Geneva: WTO. http://www.wto.org.

WWF (World Wildlife Fund). 2010. Bluefin tuna in crisis. http://www.panda.org/what_we_do/footprint/smart_fishing/sustainable_fisheries/bluefin_tuna.

Worm, B., et al. 2005. Global patterns of predator diversity in the open oceans. *Science* 309:1365–1369.

Worm, B., et al. 2006. Impacts of biodiversity loss on ocean ecosystem services. *Science* 314:787–790.

Wright, J. D., Wang, C. Y., Kennedy-Stephenson, J. and R. B. Ervin. 2003. Dietary intake of ten key nutrients for public health, United States: 1999–2000. *Advance Data from Vital and Health Statistics* 334:1–4.

Xiao, C. 2008. Health effects of soy protein and isoflavones in humans. *Journal of Nutrition* 138:1244S–1249S.

Yamada, T., et al. 2000. Atherosclerosis and ω-3 fatty acids in the populations of a fishing and a farming village in Japan. *Atherosclerosis* 153:469–481.

Yamagishi, K., et al. 2008. Fish, ω-3 polyunsaturated fatty acids, and mortality from cardiovascular diseases in a nationwide community-based cohort of Japanese men and women. *Journal of the American College of Cardiology* 52:71–79.

Yamaguchi, S., and K. Ninomiya. 2000. Umami and food palatability. *Journal of Nutrition* 130:921S–926S.

Yamamoto, T. 2007. The sweet side of Japanese cuisine. http://www.kikkoman.com/foodforum/thejapanesetable/04.shtml

Yokota, H., A. Morita, and F. Ghanati. 2005. Growth characteristics of tea plants and tea fields in Japan. *Soil Science and Plant Nutrition* 51:625–627.

Yoneda, S., and K. Hoshino. 1998. *Zen Vegetarian Cooking*. Tokyo: Kodansha International.

Yoshida, Y., Sasaki, G., Goto, S., Yanagiya, S., and K. Takashina. 1975. Studies on the etiology of milk intolerance in Japanese adults. *Journal of Gastroenterology* 10:29–34.

Yoshinaga, M., et al. 2003. Rapid increase in the prevalence of obesity in elementary school children. *International Journal of Obesity* 28:494–499.

Yoshino, M. 1986. *Sushi*. Tokyo: Gakken.

Yuge, K., M. Anan, and Y. Nakano. 2008. Historical development of rice paddy irrigation system and problems of water management in recent years: Yamada diversion dam command area in Japan. *Journal of the Faculty of Agriculture Kyushu University* 53:215–220.

Zeller, D., and D. Pauly, eds. 2007. *Reconstruction of Marine Fisheries Catches for Key Countries and Regions (1950–2005)*. Vancouver, BC: Fisheries Centre, University of British Columbia.

Zhang, J., S. Sasaki, K. Amano, and H. Kesteloot. 1999. Fish consumption and mortality from all causes, ischemic heart disease, and stroke: An ecological study. *Preventive Medicine* 28:520–529.

Zimmer, D., and D. Renault. 2003. Virtual water in food production and global trade: Review of methodological issues and preliminary results. In *Virtual Water Trade: Proceedings of the International Expert Meeting on Virtual Water Trade*, ed. A. Y. Hoekstra, 1–19. Delft: IHE (Institute for Water Education).

Index

Note: *Only the more common Japanese names of foodstuffs are indexed.*